4 Minute Keto

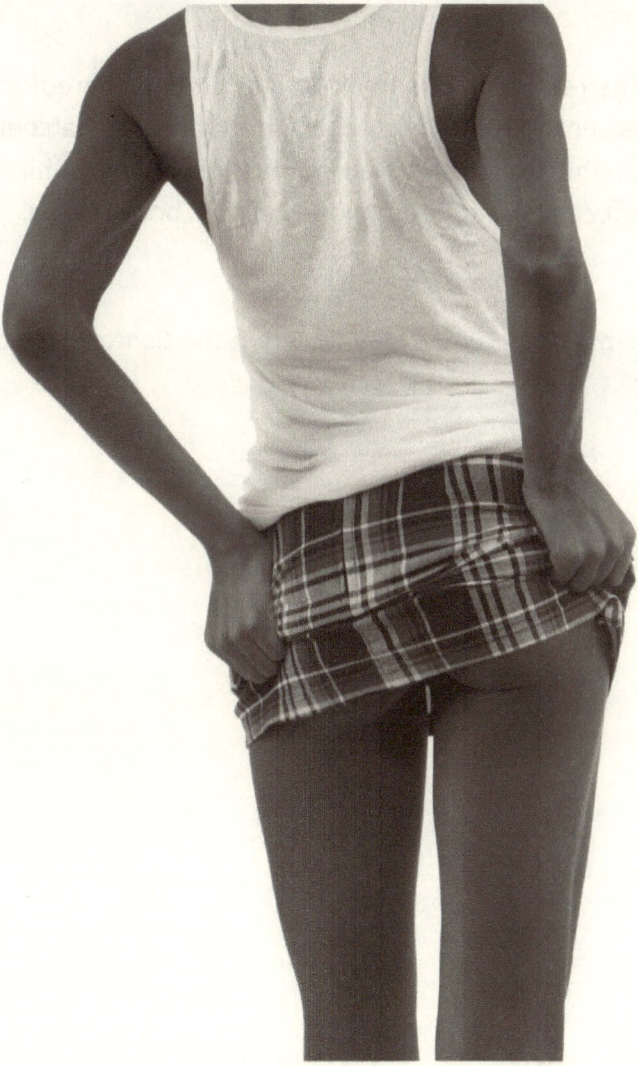

Turn your body into a lean, mean, fat-burning machine

Copyright and Enquiries

Comments or enquiries may be left in the *Contact Us* page at

https://agingslowdown.com/contact-us/

Disclaimer

Please note the information contained within this document is for educational and entertainment purposes only. Every attempt has been made to provide accurate, up to date, reliable and complete information. No warranties of any kind are expressed or implied. Readers acknowledge that the author is not engaging in the rendering of legal, financial, medical or professional advice.

By reading this document, the reader agrees that under no circumstances is the author or publisher responsible for any losses, direct or indirect, which are incurred as a result of the use of information contained within this document, including, but not limited to, errors, omissions, or inaccuracies.

Contents

4 Minute Keto

Introduction: What This Book is About

Diet and Exercise

It's no secret that the "secret" to losing weight, getting fit, resisting illness and living a long and healthy life is diet and exercise. Yet only a small proportion of the population actually put those two things into practice.

As a result, we have overwhelming rates of obesity and a generation of children who, for the first time in history have a lower life expectancy than their parents.

How bad is that?

I want you to be the exception.

And it's relatively easy.

Let's look at these two factors, diet and exercise and see what you can do about them.

Diet

I really dislike the term "diet".

Mainly because it's strayed so far from its original meaning of "what you eat."

Now, it's all about specifics – the Atkins Diet, the Paleo Diet, the Onion Soup Diet (really?) the Grapefruit Diet and so on.

Originally, I reacted in exactly the same way to the Keto diet.

But then I examined it in a little more detail.

4 Minute Keto

And discovered that, with a couple of exceptions, it was pretty much what I was eating anyway.

I'll cover the exceptions later on in this book.

Why should what I eat personally be significant anyway?

Well, it's what qualifies me to write about health and fitness.

You see, I'm 76 years old (in 2020). I bench press more than my own body weight, I can do 110 push-ups without stopping and hold a 5-minute plank. I do 100km bike rides for fun. I weigh the same as I did when I was 18 and still have the same 30" waist.

More importantly, I never get sick. Ever. No colds, no flu, no headaches, no gastric issues. And I take no drugs, prescribed or over the counter. I drink a couple of bottles of wine a week.

When I moved to where I live now, I made an appointment with a local medical practice. When the doctor asked me what the problem was, I told her I didn't have any, but I needed a doctor's name to fill in when required on various forms and could I use hers.

She was quite amused but asked if she could run a set of tests. You know, blood pressure, cholesterol, body fat etc. Everything came up fine.

And it's all down to those two things, diet and exercise.

We're going to cover the Keto diet first.

4 Minute Keto

This needs to be your way of eating.

The process is simple.

All your meals will be delicious high protein, high fat, low carb.

They'll keep your body in a state of ketosis, where instead of metabolising (burning) the glucose in your bloodstream for fuel, it will instead access your stored fat.

Your body will become a fat-burning machine.

The Keto Diet

Although the ketogenic diet has been around for almost a century, it is rapidly gaining popularity today. There is a reason why keto is so highly regarded. It's not a fad diet. It actually works, and it has tremendous health benefits in addition to weight loss. When on the keto diet, you are feeding your body exactly what it needs, while eliminating toxins that will slow it down.

The keto diet focuses on low carbohydrates, which the body converts into energy to help speed up weight loss.

What exactly is the problem with high carbs, and why should you avoid them? Carbohydrates are converted into glucose and cause a spike in insulin. The insulin enters the bloodstream to process the glucose, which then becomes the main source of energy. A spike in insulin can also result in the storage of fats. The body uses carbohydrates and fats as energy, the former being the primary source. So the more carbs you consume in your daily diet, the less fat is being burned for energy. Instead, the spike in insulin will result in more fat storage.

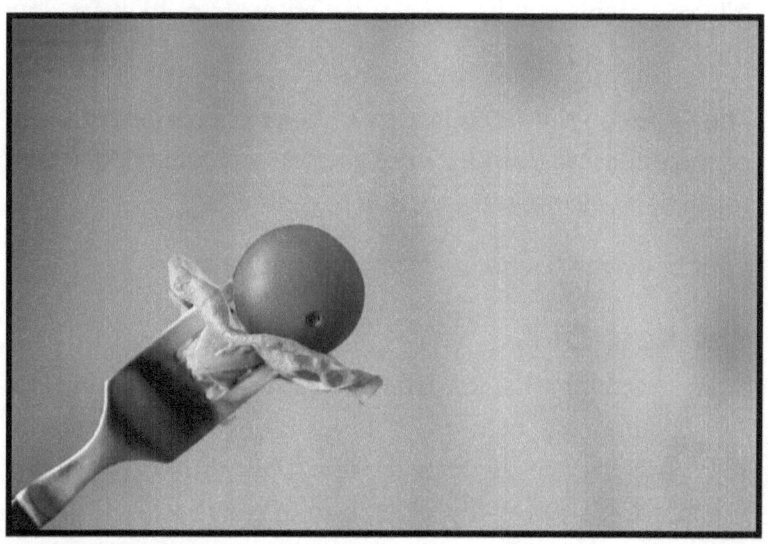

Get into a State of Ketosis

When you consume fewer carbohydrates, the body goes into a state referred to as ketosis. Thus, the name for this low-carb diet.

Ketosis helps the body survive on less food. By being in ketosis, you 'train' your body to utilize fats as the main source of energy instead of carbs, simply because there is close to zero carbs to begin with. During ketosis, the liver breaks down fats into ketones, which enables the body to use the fat as energy. During a keto diet, we don't starve ourselves of calories; we starve the body of carbohydrates. This makes weight loss easy and natural. Later on, you'll learn that the keto diet has many additional health benefits besides fat loss.

The keto diet is an easy diet, but some people do miss beans and breads. It takes a bit of getting used to. Starting anything new is challenging after all. But ultimately, you'll feel so much better, both physically and mentally that you'd be happy to avoid carbs once and for all. And being able to eat bacon on a diet does have its rewards!

We'll examine the Keto diet in detail in the next chapter.

Exercise

"It's motivation that gets us started, but habit that keeps us going."

While the Keto diet will help you lose weight by using your body's stored fat as fuel, you'll accelerate this process significantly by exercise.

And, of course, exercise will also make you look fitter and leaner, as well as feel (and be) stronger.

But most exercise programs are difficult to maintain.

You get started but stop again before it's had a chance to become a habit.

Or you just can't find the time to fit your exercise program into your daily routine.

The 4 Minute Exercise Program

That's why I developed the *4 Minute Exercise Program*.

4 Minute Keto

Turn your body into a lean, mean, fat-burning machine

It consists of a series of exercises, targeting both strength and aerobics, that take just 4 minutes to complete and require no special equipment.

The time commitment is low, but the payoff is huge.

4 Minute HIIT

HIIT stands for High Intensity Interval Training. It has been shown to be the most effective way of kick starting your body's metabolism and then keeping it burning for hours afterwards.

4 Minute Strength

This set tones and strengthens your upper and lower body musculature.

4 Minute Abs

Whether you want six pack abs or just a flat tummy, these will develop your abdominal muscles for the Keto diet to expose them.

Stretches

It's really important to stretch your muscles and increase joint mobility, particularly as you get older.

You only do one of the 4-minute workouts plus the stretches each day, so it's a minor commitment out of your busy day.

Easy, right? But the difference between doing something and doing nothing is the biggest difference of all.

4 Minute Keto

Turn your body into a lean, mean, fat-burning machine

When you're ready to ramp it up, I've got plenty of workouts to make you sweat and increase your strength. More on that later.

I'll cover the three 4 Minute sets and the stretches after looking at the Keto diet in detail.

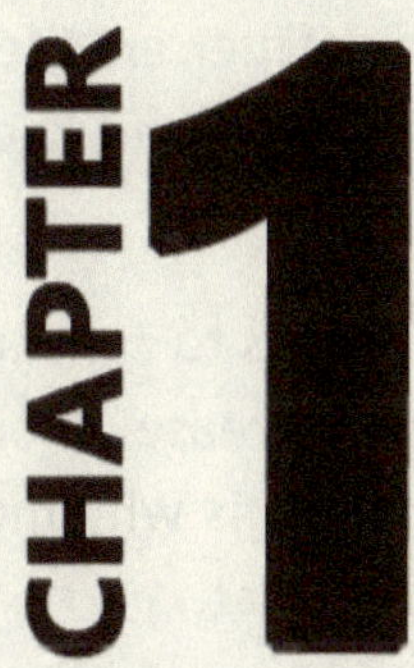

WHAT IS
KETOGENIC DIET?

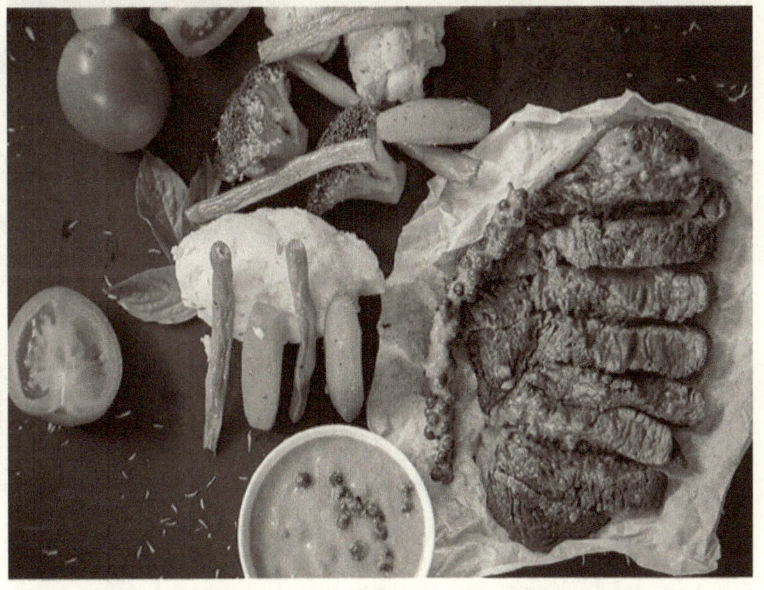

Chapter 1: What is the Ketogenic Diet?

The keto diet is a low or zero carbohydrate diet, but it differs from other low-carb diets (such as Paleo) in that it deliberately manipulates the ratios of carbs, fats, and protein to switch fat into the body's primary

4 Minute Keto

source of fuel. Our bodies are used to using carbohydrates as fuel. Fats, which are a secondary source of fuel, are rarely tapped on. That means the extra fat is stored and keeps adding on the pounds.

The only way to reduce fat in a 'normal' diet is to consume less fat and workout a lot in order to increase energy expenditure over daily calories intake, which is why most people fail to lose weight on a conventional diet.

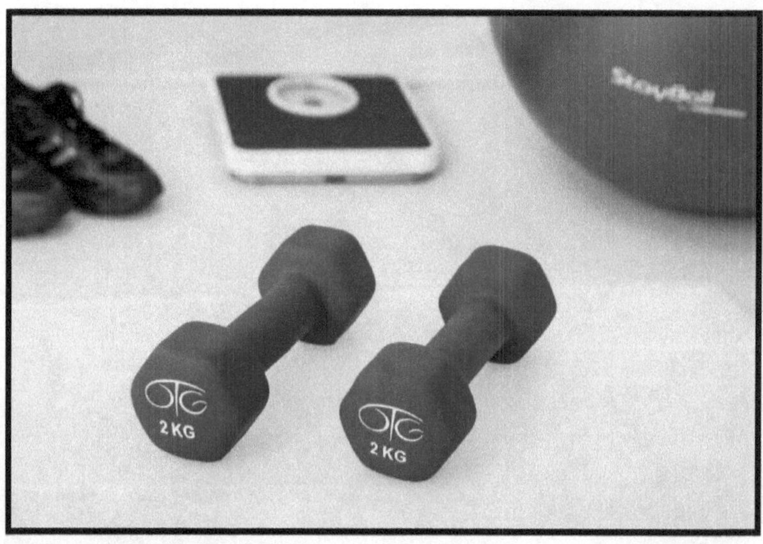

Uses Fat for Fuel

On the other hand, the ketogenic diet uses fat for fuel, which means it gets used instead of being stored. So, weight loss becomes easy. In addition to weight loss, the ketogenic diet is known as the "healing" diet. The lack of sugar intake has been proven to help and prevent many diseases such as heart disease, high blood pressure, cancers, epilepsy, and many symptoms of aging.

4 Minute Keto

The State of Ketosis

The manipulation of carbs, fats, and protein is crucial in order to get into ketosis. It's a state when the body, deprived of the usual carbohydrates and sugar, is forced to use fat as its primary fuel. So the ratio of fats and protein are significantly higher than carbs in general.

Of course, consuming less carbs also means lowering the amount of insulin in your body. Less insulin means less glucose and fat storage. That is why the keto diet has been so successful in helping people with diabetes. It adjusts the sugar level naturally.

Carbs, Fat and Protein

The ratio of carbs, fat, and protein can vary. Many people allow themselves up to 50 grams of carbohydrates a day and still lose weight. On a stricter regime, the carb intake can be between 15 and 20 grams daily. The less carbs, the quicker the weight loss, but the diet is very flexible.

On the keto diet, you don't count calories. You count carbohydrates and adjust the intake of carbs vs. fat and protein. A typical keto diet will get 60 percent of its calories from fat, 15 to 25 percent of calories from protein, and 25 percent of calories from carbohydrates. The only limitation on the diet is sugar, which you need to avoid.

Healing Effects

The ketogenic diet is not a fad. Many scientific studies have shown the benefits and healing effects of ketosis. Discuss the ketogenic diet with your doctor if you are interested in

4 Minute Keto

consuming less sugar, losing weight, or as a preventive measure against vulnerable health problems.

4 Minute Keto

Turn your body into a lean, mean, fat-burning machine

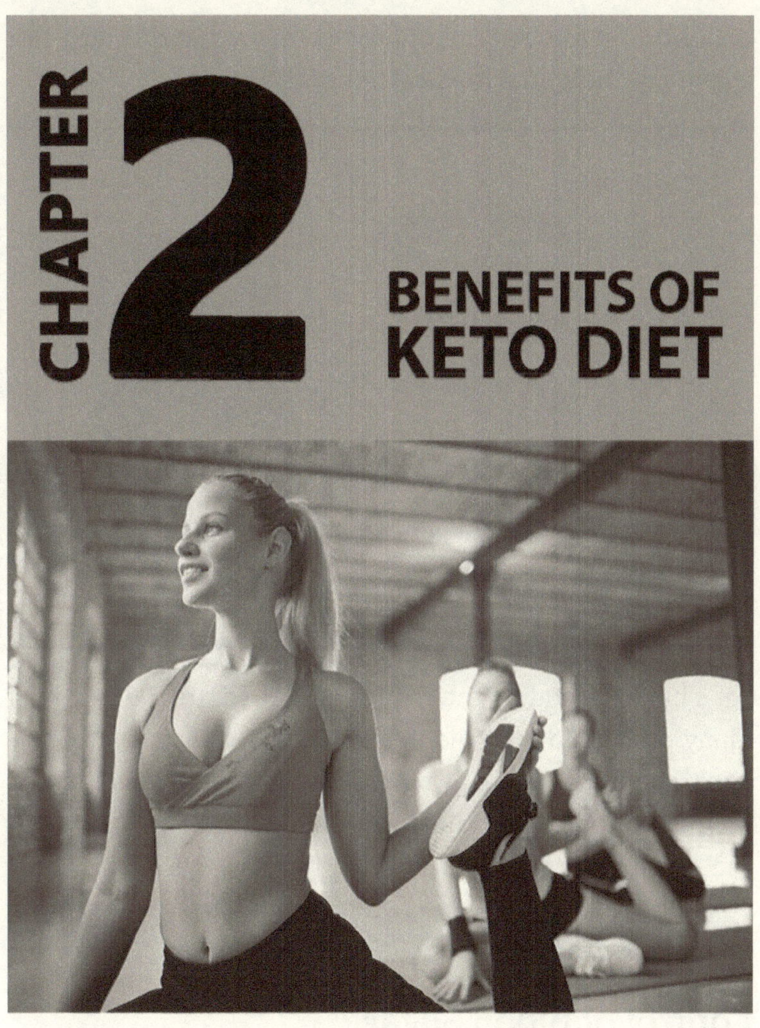

Chapter 2: Benefits of the Keto Diet

Although the ketogenic diet is popularly known as a 'rapid fat loss diet', there is actually more to this than meets the eye. In fact, weight loss and higher levels of energy are only by-products of the keto diet, a kind

4 Minute Keto

of bonus. It has been scientifically proven that the keto diet has many additional medical benefits.

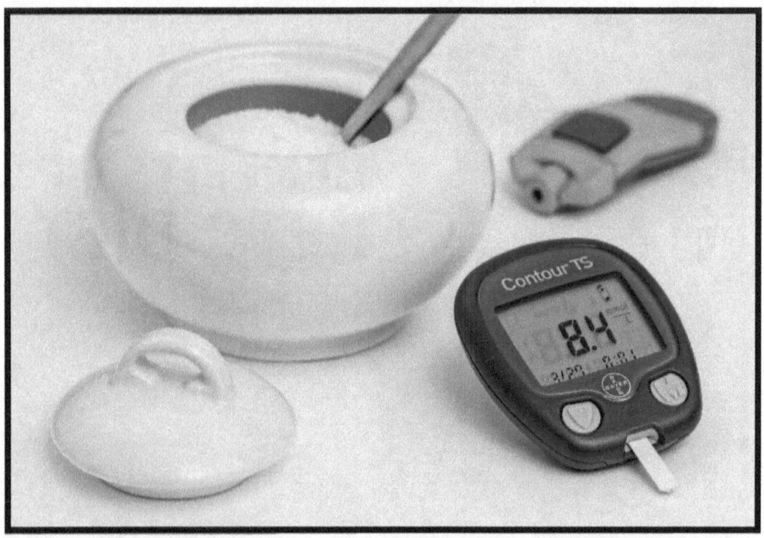

Let's begin by stating that a high carbohydrate diet, with its many processed ingredients and sugars, has absolutely no health benefits. These are merely empty calories, and most processed foods ultimately serve only to rob your body of the nutrients it needs to remain healthy. Here is a list of actual benefits for lowering your carbohydrates and eating fats that convert to energy:

Control of Blood Sugar

Keeping blood sugar at a low level is critical to manage and prevent diabetes. The keto diet has been proven to be extremely effective in preventing diabetes.

Many people suffering from diabetes are also overweight. That makes an easy weight-loss regime a natural. But the keto diet does more. Carbohydrates get converted to sugar, which for diabetics can result in a sugar spike. A diet low in carbohydrates prevents these spikes and allows more control over blood sugar levels.

Mental Focus

The keto diet is based on protein, fats, and low carbohydrates. As we've discussed, this forces fat to become the primary source of energy. This is not the normal western diet, which can be quite deficient in nutrients, particularly fatty acids, which are needed for proper brain function.

When people suffer from cognitive diseases, such as Alzheimer's, the brain isn't using enough glucose, thus becomes lacking in energy, and the brain has difficulty functioning at a high level. The keto diet provides an additional energy source for the brain.

A study by the American Diabetes Association found that Type 1 diabetics improved their brain function after consuming coconut oil.

That same study indicated that people who suffer from Alzheimer's may experience improved memory capacity on a keto diet. Those with Alzheimer's have seen improved memory scores that might correlate with the amount of ketones levels present.

What does this study mean to an average person? With the emphasis on fatty acids, such as omega 3 and omega 6 found in seafood, the keto diet is likely to fuel the brain with

4 Minute Keto

the additional nutrients to help achieve a healthier mental state. The brain tissue is made up largely of fatty acids (you've heard fish referred to as "brainfood"), and the increased consumption of those fatty acids will logically lead to improved brain health.

Our body does not produce fatty acids on its own; we can only obtain it through our diet. And the keto diet is rich in fatty acids.

A diet high in carbohydrates can lead to a "foggy" brain, where you have difficulty in focusing. Focusing becomes easier with the increased energy provided by the keto diet. In fact, many people who have no need or desire to lose weight use the keto diet to improve and enhance brain functions.

Increased Energy

It's not unusual, and has become almost normal, to feel tired and drained at the end of the day as a result of a poor, carbohydrate-laden diet. Fat is a more efficient source of energy, leaving you feeling more vitalized than you would on a "sugar" rush.

Acne

While most of the benefits of a keto diet are well-documented, one benefit catches some people by surprise: better skin and less acne. Acne is fairly common. Ninety percent of teens suffer from it, and many adults do, as well.

While it was always thought that acne was at least exacerbated by poor diet, controlled research is still being conducted. However, many people on the keto diet have reported clearer skin. There may be a logical reason. A 1972 study found that high levels of insulin can cause the eruption of acne. Since a keto diet keeps insulin at a low and healthy level, it may very well affect skin health.

In addition, acne thrives on inflammation. The ketogenic diet eases and reduces inflammation, thus enabling the body to decrease acne eruptions. Fatty acids, which are found in abundance in fish, are a known anti-inflammatory.

While research is still being done, it seems likely that a keto diet has beneficial effects for clearer, healthier, more glowing skin.

Keto and Anti-Aging

Many diseases are a natural result of the aging process. While there have not been studies done on humans, studies on mice have shown brain cell improvement on a keto diet.

Several studies have shown a positive effect of the keto diet on patients with Alzheimer's disease. What we do know is that a diet filled with good nutrients and antioxidants, low in sugar, high in protein and healthy fats, while low in carbohydrates, enhances our overall health. It protects us from the toxins of a poor diet.

There is also research indicating that using fatty acids for fuel instead of sugar may slow down the aging process, possibly because of the negative effects that sugar has on our overall wellbeing.

4 Minute Keto

In addition, the simple act of eating less and consuming fewer calories is a matter of basic health, as it prevents obesity and its inherent side effects.

So far, studies have been limited. However, considering the powerful positive effects of the ketogenic diet on our health, it is logical to assume this diet will help us grow older in a more natural way while delaying the natural effect of aging. A normal western diet laden with sugars and processed foods are certainly detrimental to warding off the signs of aging.

Keto and Hunger

One of the major reasons diets fail is hunger. People who diet feel hungry and deprived and simply give up. A low carbohydrate diet naturally leaves people feeling full and satisfied. Less hungry means people will actually remain on the diet longer while consuming fewer calories.

Keto and Eyesight

Diabetics are aware that high blood sugar can lead to a higher risk of developing cataracts. Since the keto diet controls sugar levels, it can help retain eyesight and help prevent cataracts. This has been proven in several studies involving diabetic patients.

Keto and Autism

We know the keto diet affects brain functions. In a study on autism, it was found that it also has a positive effect on autism. Thirty autistic children were placed on the keto diet. All showed improvement in autistic behavior, especially

4 Minute Keto

those on the milder autistic spectrum. While more studies are needed, the results were extremely positive.

4 Minute Keto

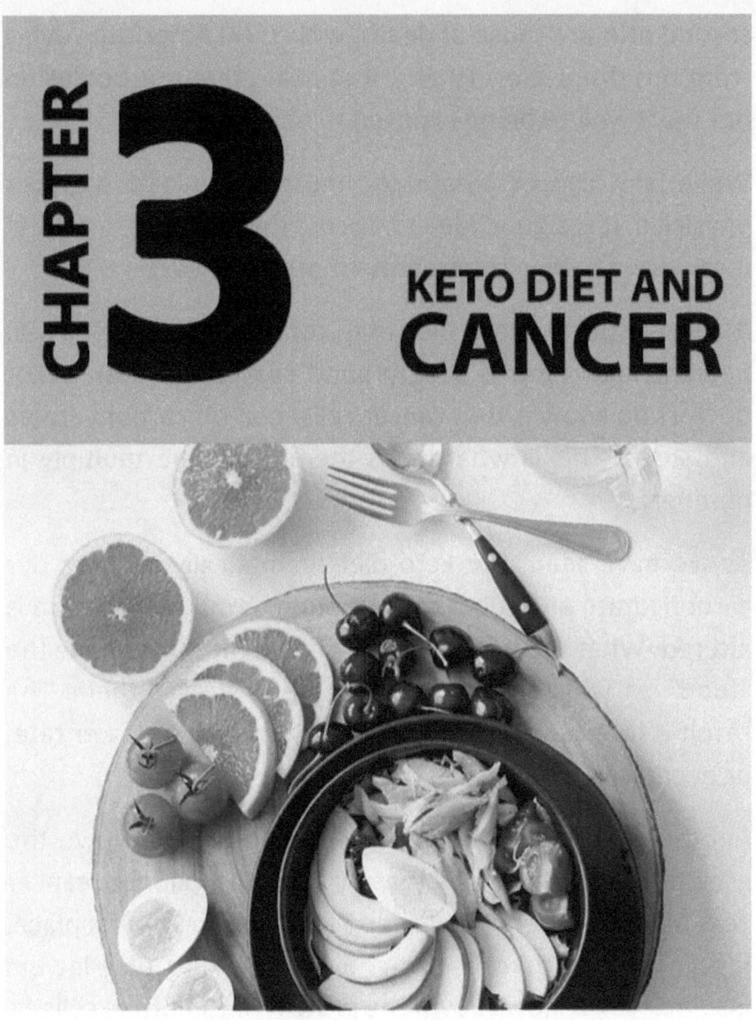

Chapter 3: Keto Diet and Cancer

Cancer has turned into a serious disease in our modern society. While cancer was not a large factor before the 20th century (it did exist, of course), our modern diet and sedentary lifestyle have made cancer the second primary cause of death, with 1600 Americans dying from this disease every day. It appears that our bodies do not react well to being exposed to daily toxins.

While any cancer treatment must be guided by your physician, it is a good idea to discuss the keto diet and what it can do to help in the treatment of this disease.

A cancer-specific keto diet may consist of as much as 90 percent fat. There is a very good reason for that. What doctors do know is that cancer cells feed off carbohydrates and sugar. This is what helps them grow and multiply in number.

As we have seen, the keto diet dramatically reduces our carbohydrate and sugar consumption as our metabolism is altered. What the keto diet does, in essence, is remove the "food" on which cancer cells feed and starves them. The result is that cancer cells may die, multiply at a slower rate, or decrease.

Another reason why a keto diet is able to slow down the growth of cancer cells is that by reducing calories, cancer cells have less energy to develop and grow in the first place. Insulin also helps cells grow. Since the keto diet lowers insulin level, it slows down the growth of tumorous cells.

When on the keto diet, the body produces ketones. While the body is fueled by ketones, cancerous cells are not. Therefore, a state of ketosis may help reduce the size and growth of cancer cells.

4 Minute Keto

One study monitored the growth of tumors in patients suffering from cancer of the digestive tract. Of those patients who received a high carbohydrate diet, tumors showed a 32.2 percent in growth. Patients on a keto diet showed a 24.3 percent growth in their tumor. The difference is significant.

Another study involved five patients who combined chemotherapy with a keto diet. Three of these patients went into remission. Two patients saw a progression of the disease when they went off the keto diet.

More studies are needed, but these numbers are encouraging.

The keto diet may help prevent cancer from occurring in diabetic patients in the first place. People with diabetes have a higher risk level to develop cancer due to elevated blood sugar levels. Since the ketogenic diet is extremely effective at decreasing the levels of blood sugar, it may prevent the initial onset of cancer.

4 Minute Keto

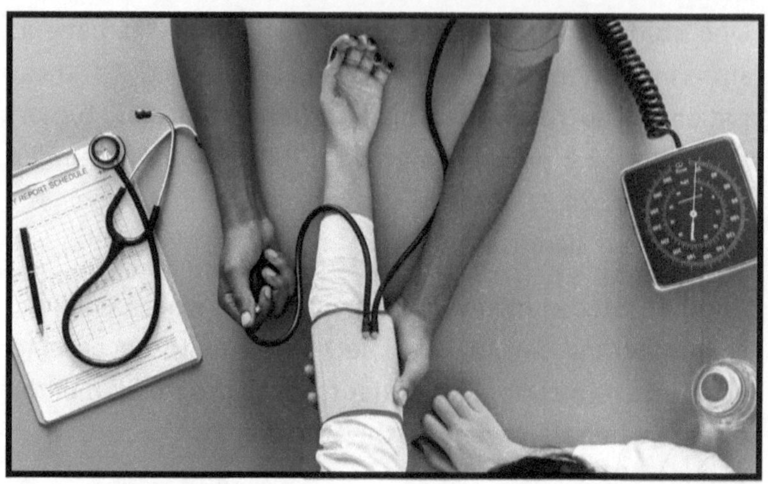

From what research has discovered so far, a ketogenic diet may:

1. Stop the growth of cancer cells.

2. Help replace cancerous cells with healthy cells.

3. Change the body's metabolism and enable the body to "starve" cancer cells by depriving them of needed nutrition.

4. By lowering the body's insulin level, the ketogenic body may prevent the onset of cancer cells.

On a ketogenic diet specifically for cancer, your fats should be 75 to 90 percent, protein 15-20 percent, and less than 5 percent carbohydrates.

Foods to Eat

1. Egg, including yolks

4 Minute Keto

Turn your body into a lean, mean, fat-burning machine

2. All green, leafy vegetables, as well as cauliflower, avocado, mushrooms, peppers, cucumbers, and tomatoes.

3. When choosing dairy, opt for full-fat versions of cheese, butter, sour cream, yogurt, and milk.

4. Eat nuts such as walnuts, almonds, filberts, and sunflower and pumpkin seeds.

Foods to Eat in Moderation

1. Have one serving of root vegetables, such as yams, parsnip, carrots or turnips per day.

2. Fruits contain sugar, so treat them like candy. One small piece per day.

3. A glass of dry wine, vodka, whiskey or brandy once a week. No cocktails with sugars.

4. A small piece of chocolate with 75 percent or higher cocoa content once a week.

Foods to Avoid

1. Any food containing sugar, including cereals; soft drinks, juices, and sports drinks, candies, and chocolate. Limit artificial sweeteners as much as possible.

2. Starchy food such as pasta and potatoes, breads, potato chips, french fries, cooking oils (other than coconut and extra virgin olive oil) and margarine.

3. All beers.

4 Minute Keto

Turn your body into a lean, mean, fat-burning machine

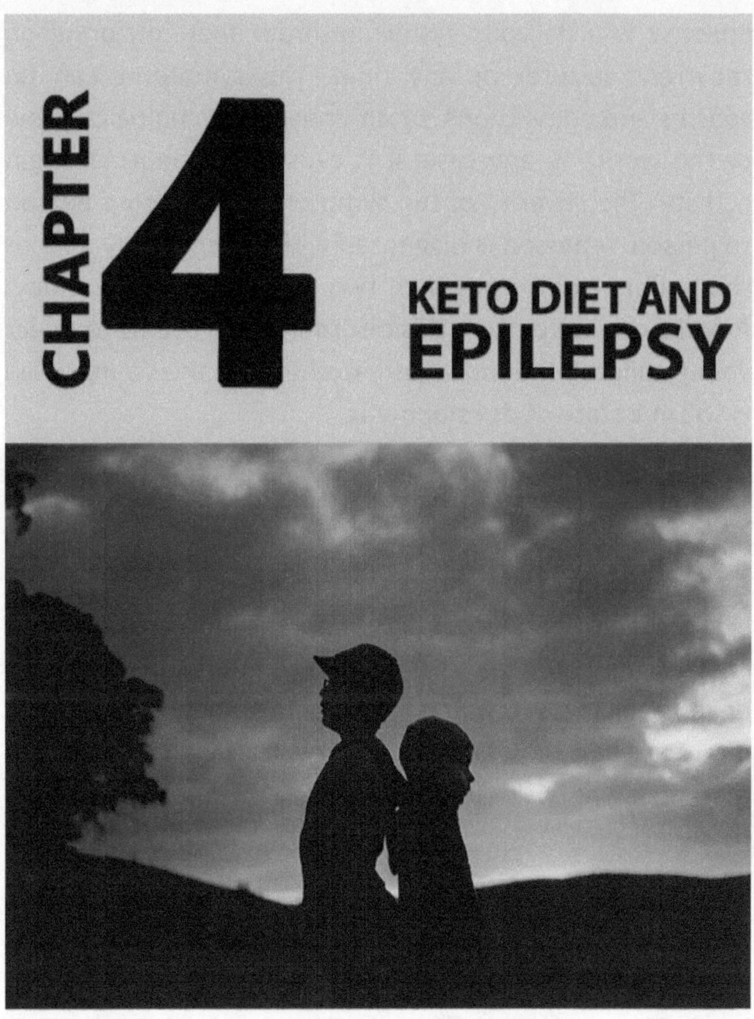

Chapter 4: Keto Diet and Epilepsy

The initial use of the keto diet had nothing to do with weight loss or diabetes management, for which it is now so well-known. Instead, the diet was created by a doctor in 1924 to help his patients suffering from epilepsy.

4 Minute Keto

Epilepsy is a nervous system disorder that can bring on recurrent seizures at any time. The symptoms can be spasms and convulsions, or an unusual psychological view of the world. In any case, it is caused by abnormal brain activity. The severity of the symptoms varies from person to person. A person is diagnosed with epilepsy only if he or she suffers from more than two seizures in one full day. Anyone can suffer from this disorder, but it seems to affect young children the most, perhaps because the young brain is still in a state of development.

Seizures are frequently managed by drugs. Sometimes they work and sometimes they don't.

As far back as 1924, however, Dr. Russell Wilder of the Mayo Clinic conducted groundbreaking research and created the ketogenic diet to help children suffering from epilepsy. It was remarkably effective, but doctors lost interest when new anti-seizure medications came on the market. It was easier for them to prescribe medication than to discuss diet.

However, people who used the keto diet to treat seizures continued seeing remarkable success. Today, doctors are returning to using the low carbohydrate, high-fat diet to treat their patients. The results have been extremely promising.

In 1998, the Journal of Pediatrics published a study involving 150 children who experienced seizures despite taking popular anti-seizure medications. The children were

4 Minute Keto

placed on the ketogenic diet for one year which the researchers assessed their progress.

Eighty-three percent of the subjects were still in the study after 3 months. Over one-third of the children showed a 90 percent decrease in seizures. At the end of the year, slightly more than half of the subjects had remained on the diet, and a quarter of them experienced a 90 percent decrease in seizures. The numbers indicate that the keto diet has a tremendously positive effect on children who suffer from seizures. The researchers consider it more effective than medication in many cases.

For anyone with children who experience seizures, the inclusion of a keto diet in the child's treatment should be discussed with his or her physician.

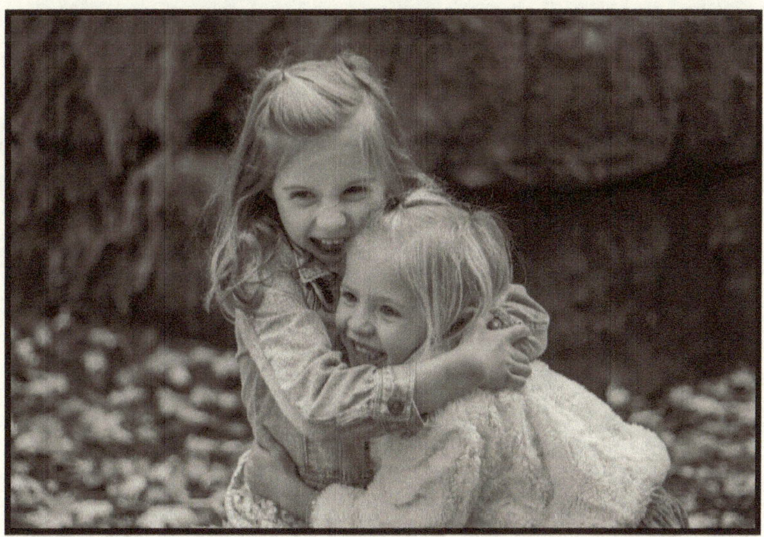

Another research on the effects of the keto diet on childhood epilepsy involved 145 children. The children were divided into two groups, with one group being treated with medication while the other group receiving a ketogenic diet. Seventy-four percent of the ketogenic diet group were successful in reducing seizures.

There have been more studies of childhood epilepsy and the keto diet. These have sparked new and considerable interest within the medical profession.

4 Minute Keto

Turn your body into a lean, mean, fat-burning machine

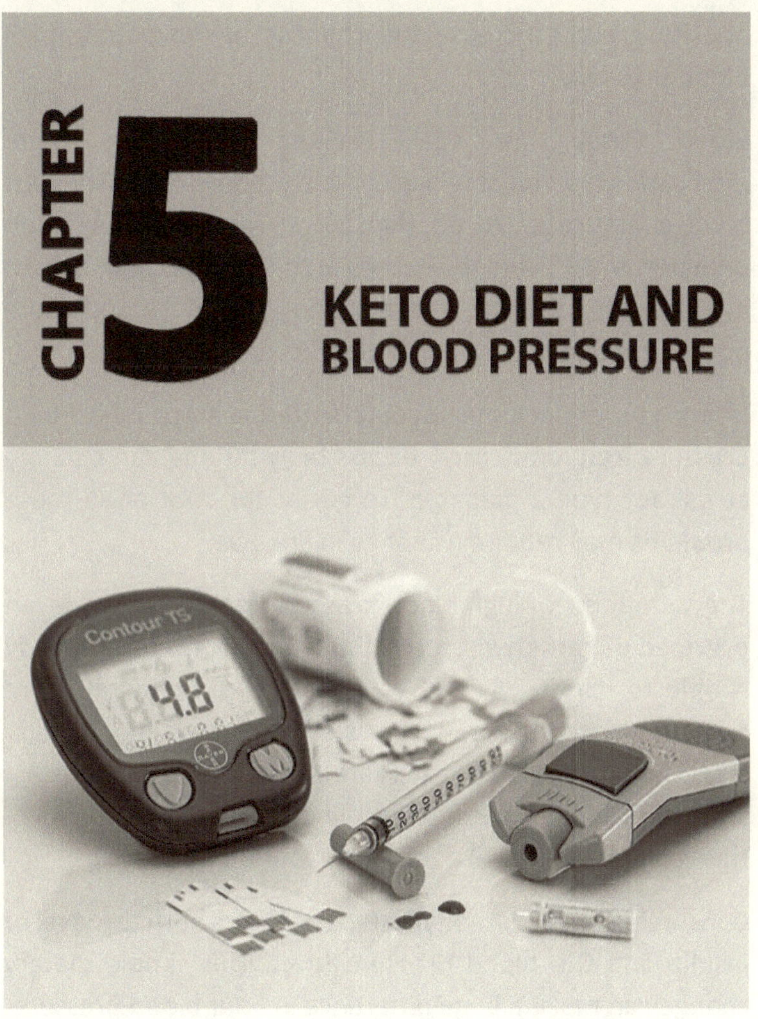

Chapter 5: Keto Diet and Blood Pressure

One-third of American adults suffer from high blood pressure. It is a serious health problem that can lead to heart attacks and strokes. Obviously, the higher the blood pressure, the greater the risk. Aging and obesity greatly increase the chances of developing high blood pressure.

Blood pressure is usually treated with a variety of medications, some of which can have side effects. The best blood pressure is 120/80. High blood pressure is the result of hypertension, and the causes aren't always clear, but we live in an increasingly tense world, and more and more people are dealing with high blood pressure.

It is a known fact that people suffering from high blood pressure frequently carry excess belly fat and can become at risk for type 2 diabetes. To get at the root of all these problems may require a change in lifestyle.

The symptoms of high blood pressure can be caused by an overload of carbohydrates in the diet, more than the body is able to handle. As we've discussed, carbohydrates are converted into sugars, which raise the body's blood sugar level, forcing the body to create additional insulin. Insulin stores fat, and an excess of insulin can lead to obesity. All of this can have a negative effect on your blood pressure.

Consuming fewer carbohydrates decreases both the level of insulin and the blood pressure level. This simple dietary change can make a huge difference in your blood pressure.

In an interesting study released in the Archives of Internal Medicine, 146 overweight people took part in a weight-loss experiment. The people were divided into two groups. One group was put on a ketogenic diet containing a maximum of 20 grams of carbohydrates, while the other group was given

4 Minute Keto

the weight-loss drug orlistat, in addition to being counseled to follow a low-fat regimen.

Both groups showed similar weight loss. What surprised the researchers was that half of the keto group showed a decrease in blood pressure, while only 21 percent of the low-fat diet group had any decrease in blood pressure. While weight loss itself would bring about a lowering of blood pressure, the study suggests that a decrease in carbohydrate intake can help lower blood pressure even more.

It was found that potassium specifically had a huge effect on lower hypertension. Doctors recommend at least 4,700 mg of potassium each day for anyone wishing to lower his or her blood pressure.

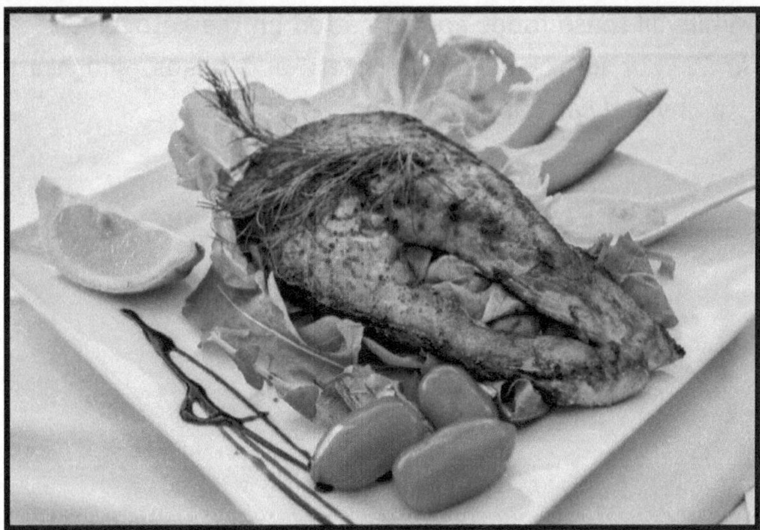

Foods high in potassium are:

4 Minute Keto

- Avocado

- Acorn squash

- Bananas

- Coconut water

- Dried apricots

- Pomegranate

- Salmon

- Spinach

- Sweet potato

- White beans

While all these foods are permitted on the ketogenic diet, limit your intake of sweet potato and beans, which are starchy and can contain a high level of carbs.

4 Minute Keto

Turn your body into a lean, mean, fat-burning machine

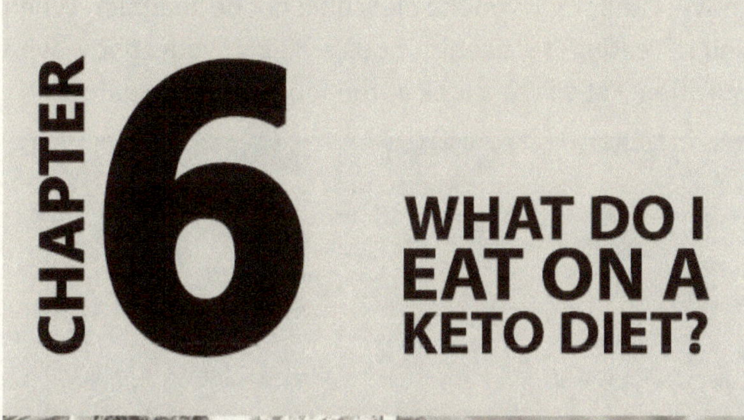

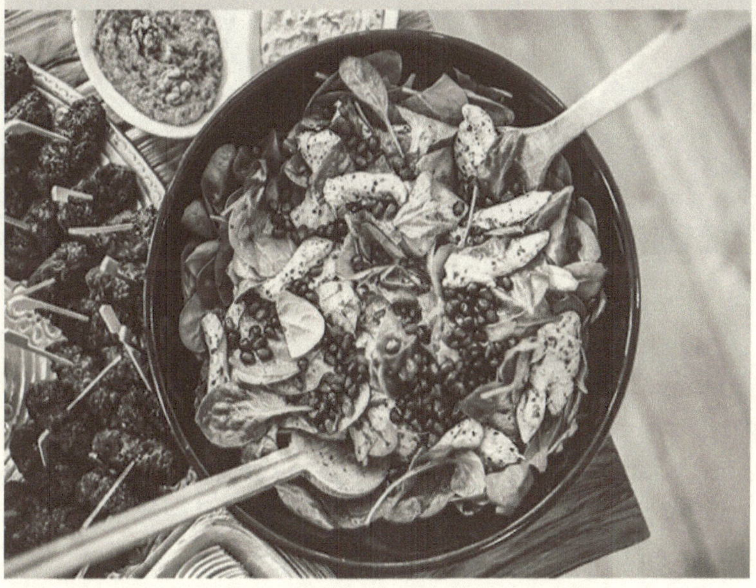

Chapter 6: What Do I Eat on a Keto Diet?

Some people associate the keto diet with the bad word "fat," and are quick to dismiss it. Nothing could be further from the truth. Fat *is* allowed, because it is converted into energy. Our body needs healthy fats to

4 Minute Keto

thrive. Other foods on the diet could not be healthier. When you're eating ketogenic, you're filling your body with nutrition. Let's take a look at the foods you'll be eating.

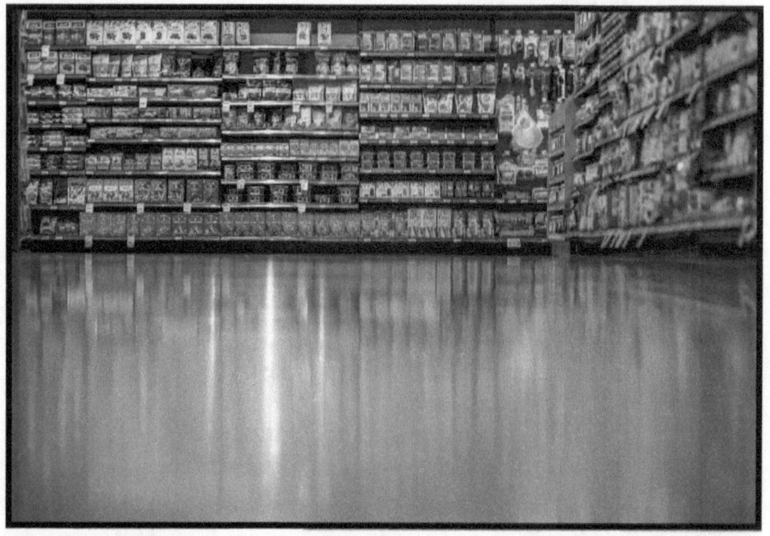

As this book has already pointed out, the elimination of processed foods and sugar is one of the best things you can do for your health in general. Processed foods are filled with toxic preservatives that do nothing for you but rob you of your good health. Fresh is always better. When purchasing anything at the market, get into the habit of reading labels. They can be very sneaky and revealing.

A useful rule of thumb when looking at food labels in the supermarket is "the fewer ingredients the better". For example, an egg's ingredients list is: eggs. Compare that with the list of stuff included in your typical cereal or TV dinner.

4 Minute Keto

Keep your carbohydrates under 50 grams a day, and you'll feel the difference. A stricter ketogenic diet will contain approximately 20 grams of carbs a day.

Food to Eat on a Ketogenic Diet

1. Seafood

Everyone knows about the healthy fatty acids, vitamins and minerals in seafood. Very few of us eat enough. The keto diet encourages the consumption of all things from the sea. Shrimp and crabs are carb-free, and other shellfish contain only a low amount of carbohydrates.

Fatty fish, such as salmon and sardines, are highly recommended because of their high omega-fatty acid content. Fish truly is brainfood. Enjoy at least two servings or more of seafood a week on the keto diet. Simple canned tuna counts as seafood.

2. Vegetables

Can a diet that recommends unlimited green, leafy vegetables be anything but healthy? They are extremely low in carbohydrates and bursting with vitamins, antioxidants, and the fiber we need daily. Green vegetables such as broccoli, spinach, and kale are believed to decrease the risk of heart diseases and cancer. Cauliflower and turnips can be prepared to look and taste like rice or mashed potatoes, with much less starch and carbohydrates.

"Starchy" vegetables, such as potatoes or beets do have carbs and should be limited on the keto diet.

4 Minute Keto

3. Dairy Foods

a.   There are cheeses to satisfy everyone's taste. They are high in fat content for energy, high in protein and calcium, and low in carbohydrates.

b.   Yogurt and cottage cheese are a great source of protein and calcium. They are low-carb and fit well into the ketogenic lifestyle. Be sure to stick with plain yogurt, as the flavored types contain a lot of sugar, as do the so-called "low fat" versions of yogurt. You can flavor yogurt and cottage cheese yourself with a few berries and nuts.

4. Avocados

Avocados are truly "superfood." They are high in important vitamins and minerals, including potassium. According to a study, avocados are also believed to help lower cholesterol by 22 percent.

Loaded with nutrients and delicious taste, avocados only have 2 grams of net carbohydrates. Use them in salads and sandwiches.

5. Meat and Poultry

The keto diet lets you eat plenty of meat. Meat contains very few carbs and is high in protein to help you build muscles. Whenever possible, choose healthy, grass-fed meats, which are higher in fatty acids.

6. Eggs

Eggs are high in protein and contain a mere 1 gram of carbohydrates. As they are also inexpensive, they are ideal for anyone on a ketogenic diet.

Eggs also make you feel full, thereby helping you eat less. Many people take pride in only consuming the whites of eggs, but the true nutrition lies in the yolk, so be sure to eat the egg in its entirety.

7. Coconut Oil

Too many people are unfamiliar with coconut oil, another "superfood." It is perfect for people dealing with diabetes and has been used with Alzheimer patients.

Coconut oil can be used in most recipes in place of butter or oil. You can also use it for frying and sautéing.

8. Dark Chocolate

Did you know that dark chocolate has high amounts of antioxidants? As a matter of fact, dark chocolate is reaching superfood status. Chocolate with 80 percent or higher real cocoa powder can lower your blood pressure.

An ounce of 80 percent dark chocolate contains 10 grams of carbohydrates, so it definitely counts as a healthy snack. Keep in mind the lower the cocoa content, the less healthy the chocolate will be. Milk chocolate does not count as a healthy chocolate.

Foods to Avoid on a Ketogenic Diet

The keto diet has a lot fewer restricted foods than many other diets. Sugar, of course, should be avoided. That doesn't mean you can't enjoy sweet desserts. There are many keto-friendly recipes that substitute unsweetened apple sauce for sugar in baked goods. Substitute sweeteners such as Stevia can also be used in moderation.

4 Minute Keto

Keep in mind that fruits are healthful, but they do contain a great deal of sugar, so limit the amount you eat to just a few slices a day. Fruit juices are concentrates that have vitamins but lack fiber. And their sugar content is extremely high. Read the label on any bottle of juice before buying. The best juices are "green" with just a hint of fruit for flavoring.

Be careful with cereals. Most are packed with sugar and robbed of any nutrients. Many claim, "nutrition added," but all that means is that all nutrition has been removed and replaced with a small amount, and a whole lot of sugar for taste. One hundred percent bran cereal will fit into your keto diet, and you can sweeten it with a handful of berries. Just be sure to examine all labels in the cereal aisle. They can be very tricky. Also, remember that honey, too, is considered as sugar.

Totally omit white starches from your diet. They are nothing but empty calories. This includes white bread, pasta, and rice. Buy the wholegrain version, instead, and enjoy in moderation.

Legumes such as beans are healthy for you, but they are high in carbohydrates. You can have them occasionally; just make sure you keep it within your daily 20 – 5o carb-gram count.

Alcohols tend to be empty calories, but certain spirits will be better for you than others. Beer is filled with carbs and should be off your keto diet. The expression "beer belly" exists for a reason. Enjoy a glass of wine, instead. Of course, there are variances in different types wine. Dry wines

4 Minute Keto

contain a minimum amount of sugar, while sweet dessert wines contain much more.

Pure alcohol such as whiskey and vodka are carb-free, but they do contain calories, so have a care. Mixing alcohol for fancy cocktails usually creates a haven for sugar, so avoid those.

Wine coolers may be a tasty treat, but in reality, they are just sugary sodas with some added alcohol. They should definitely not be on your keto diet at any time.

4 Minute Keto

Turn your body into a lean, mean, fat-burning machine

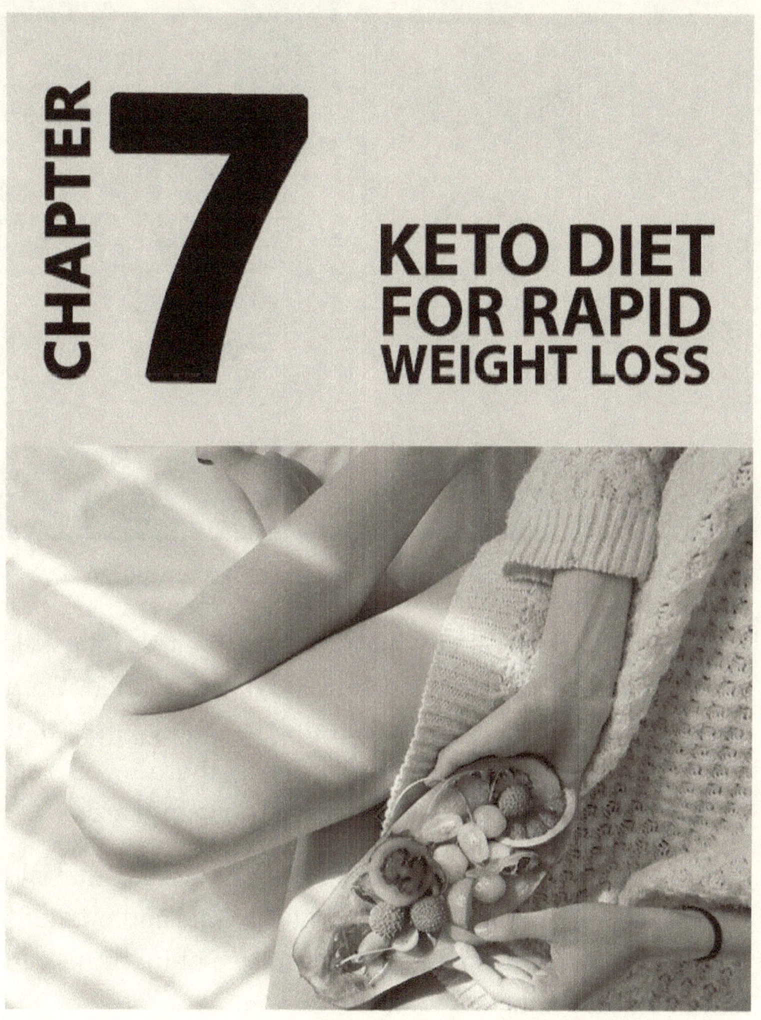

Chapter 7: Keto Diet for Rapid Weight Loss

Many people confuse the ketogenic diet with low carb diets or paleo diets. However, there are considerable differences of which you should be aware.

4 Minute Keto

Turn your body into a lean, mean, fat-burning machine

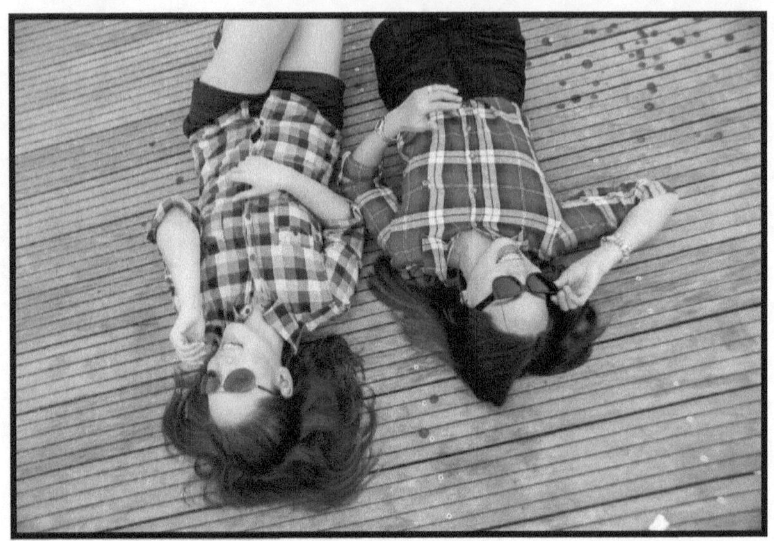

Keto v. Low Carb

A low-carb diet can be anything it wants to be, as long as it is low in carbohydrates. And "low" is rarely defined. On a low-carb diet, you simply make random food choices that curb your carb intake arbitrarily. Since there is no real number, you might still be consuming too many carbs.

Most importantly, what the low-carb diet lacks is that all-critical ketonic state that turns carbs into fats and provides your body with a new and effective source of fuel. This can leave you very hungry and tired.

The ketogenic diet has a specific ratio of carbs to fats to protein. This manipulation is critical, and it's why a low-carb diet won't work as well, if at all.

4 Minute Keto

Turn your body into a lean, mean, fat-burning machine

Keto v. Paleo

The Paleo is also a low-carb type diet. It is based on the assumption that eating the way our cavemen ancestors did, i.e., meat and no carbs, sugars, or grains, is the healthiest type of diet.

There are problems with this reasoning. First, our ancestors never experienced the kind of diseases that we face. The ketogenic diet is specifically a "healing" diet that is meant to benefit the body in many ways and help prevent diseases. The paleo diet does not do that.

Also, the paleo diet is based on eating meat instead of manipulating the ratio of fats, carbohydrates, and protein to achieve a ketonic state that uses fat as fuel.

Ketogenic Diet

Basically, ketogenic is low-carb, but it is much more.

There is a reason the ketogenic diet has become so popular. It helps improve your overall wellbeing in addition to helping you lose weight. You have more energy during the day, and you feel sated and full, thereby reducing the cravings for unhealthy snacks. In essence, you are eating less, but better. That's what makes the keto diet so unique and successful.

The ketogenic diet is not a magic pill made up by some gurus. Countless studies and testimonials are able to back the effectiveness of this diet. It is a scientifically proven method that balances your body's fat intake to help achieve optimal weight loss.

4 Minute Keto

By using fat instead of sugar as your primary source of energy, the keto diet induces a state of ketosis, which is achieved when your body stops receiving carbohydrates to turn into glucose. The fewer carbohydrates you consume, the more you force your body to burn fat for energy instead of storing it.

This is why it is possible to lose weight so quickly on the keto diet. It counts carbohydrates instead of calories. Using fats as an additional energy source is what ketosis is all about. It is a natural state that helped our hunter-gatherer ancestors survive in the early days.

They feasted on low-carb foods when they could, and fasted when food was scarce. Fat was stored and converted into energy during the scarce times. The ketogenic state is a natural human state, which makes the ketogenic diet so powerful and successful. In addition to the benefits of the keto diet, most people simply enjoy the way it makes them feel better.

Weight loss results on the keto diet differ among individuals, depending on their specific body composition. But weight loss has been the consistent result of people who've been on the keto diet. The keto diet is known as the best weight-loss diet, as well as the healthiest.

A 2017 study divided CrossFit-training subjects into two groups, with both groups following the physical training, but only one group combined the ketogenic diet with the training. The results showed that those on the keto diet decreased their fat mass and weight far more than the other group.

The keto diet group showed an average of 3.5 kilo weight loss, 2.6 percent of body fat, and 2.83 kilos in fat mass, while the other group lost no weight, body fat or fat mass. Both groups showed similar athletic performance ability.

A 2012 study divided overweight children and adolescents into two group; one was put on a keto diet, the other on a low-calorie diet. As in other keto studies, the children on the keto diet decreased their weight, fat mass, and lowered their insulin levels considerably more than the low-calorie group.

Besides more rapid weight loss, a decided advantage of the keto diet over a low-calorie diet is that people actually stick to the keto diet. A low-calorie diet will help you lose weight, but you may be constantly feeling hungry and deprived. That is the main reason most diets fail. Hunger and deprivation are not a part of the ketogenic lifestyle.

Ketosis Explained

As we have stated earlier, the keto diet isn't magic. It is proven science. Ketosis is a natural occurrence that happens when you don't feed your body enough carbohydrates and it is forced to look for energy elsewhere.

You have undoubtedly experienced ketosis when you've missed a meal or have exhausted your body with rigorous exercise. Whenever these things happen, your body helps you out by raising its level of ketones. However, most

4 Minute Keto

people eat enough sugar and carbs to keep ketosis from happening.

We love our sugar and carbs, no matter how bad they are for us, and our bodies will happily use them as fuel. And since our bodies want to help us out, it turns any excess glucose into fat and stores it for future use. Stored fat translated into that awful belly fat that you never want.

The more you restrict your carbohydrate consumption, the more your body will produce ketones. It really has no other options. When we restrict the amount of carbohydrates that we eat, our body will still provide us with energy, but it must turn to another source. And that alternate source is fat that was so thoughtfully stored for emergencies. The result is a state of ketosis. It happens when our body breaks down the fat into fatty acids and glycerol.

Researchers have discovered most of what they know about ketosis from people who fast, thereby depriving them of all sources of energy. After two days of fasting, the body is starting to produce ketones as it breaks down the available protein and begins to use stored fat for fuel. Ketosis is the natural process the body goes through when deprived of other sources of energy.

Obviously, going on a ketogenic diet is healthier than fasting. Ketogenic should become a lifestyle, not a quick weight-loss method. One of the reasons it is so beneficial is that ketones offer protection against diseases and damages that can affect the body. As mentioned before, the keto diet

4 Minute Keto

is an excellent tool to prevent many diseases and maintain health and strength longer.

Planning your keto meals will depend largely on your goals. Are you trying to lose weight, or are you on the keto diet to alleviate the symptoms of some disease? The average keto diet will consist of four meals per day, with a total of 100 grams of protein, 25-50 grams of carbohydrates, and 140-160 grams of fat. This can, of course, be adjusted to your personal needs.

For example, if you are on a keto diet to improve cognitive functions, you may want to raise your fat intake to 90 grams a day for optimal results.

Benefits of Intermittent Fasting on Keto

The science behind the ketogenic diet is that the body burns fat when deprived of other sources of fuel. Intermittent fasting is a deliberate deprivation of food and takes the concept a step further. We're not talking long-term fasting.

Intermittent fasting while on a keto diet means having two meals a day or fasting for one day a week. The fasting time gives the body a chance to rest and rid itself of toxins. It provides an extra boost to the weight-loss benefits of keto and is a great way to jump-start the diet. For weight loss, the keto diet, combined with intermittent fasting, will help you reach your goal faster and easier.

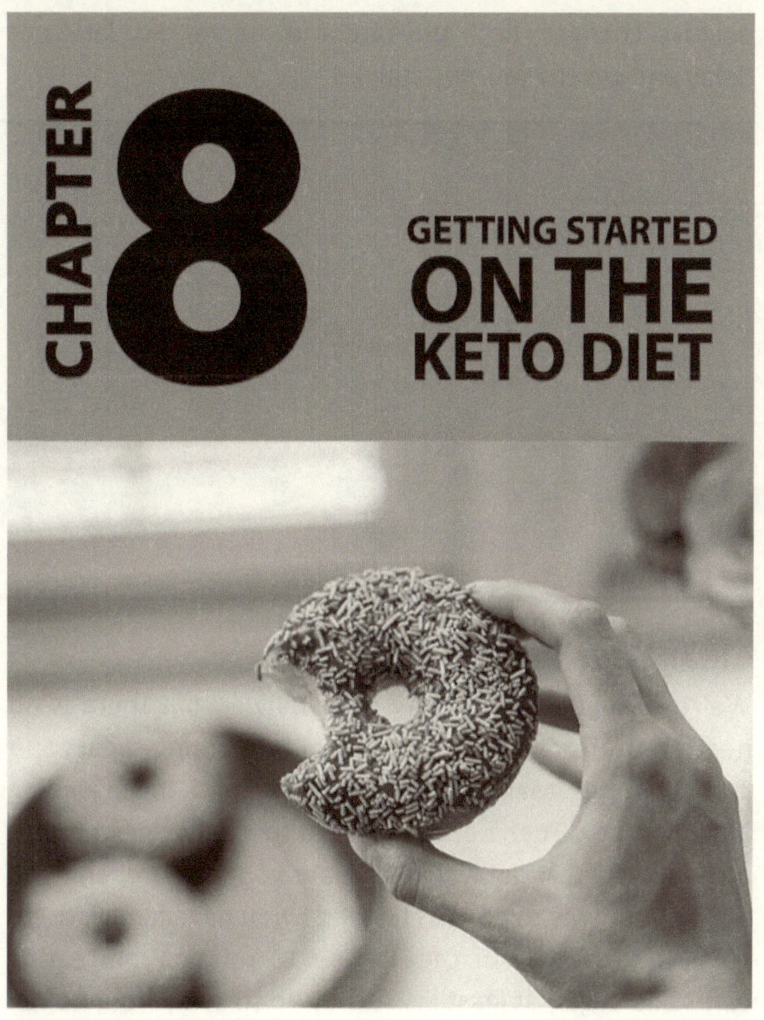

Chapter 8: Getting Started on the Keto Diet

You're ready for a new and improved you. Congratulations. There are so many wonderful benefits to the ketogenic diet, you can expect many

4 Minute Keto

positive changes, both physical and mental. So, let's not delay and get the journey started.

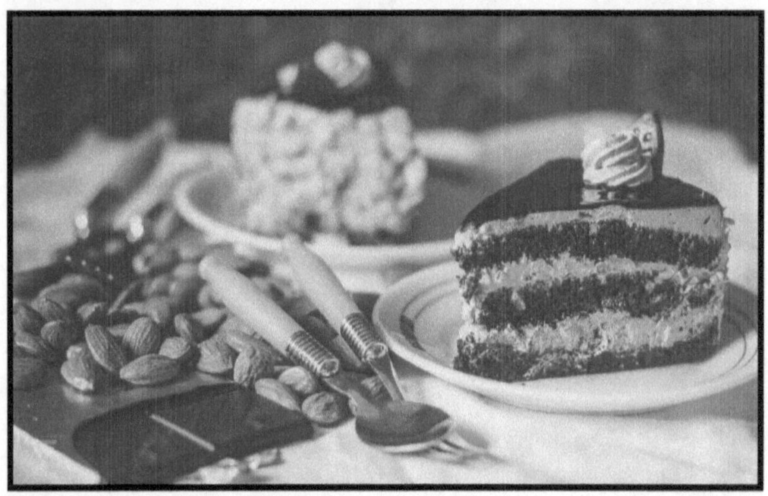

Clear Your Pantry

We're sure you have plenty of willpower, but there is no need to confront a kitchen filled with tempting sugars and carbohydrates. Make a clean sweep and pack the offending items in a box. Then donate the loot to a needy neighbor or a soup kitchen. They will appreciate your gesture, and you are on your way to a keto lifestyle. If you have family, try to get them involved. If they refuse to refrain from eating carbs and sugar, at least insist they do so away from home. It's a fair request.

Weigh Yourself

The keto diet does not require you to live by the tyranny of the scale. As a matter of fact, as you build up healthy muscles, you might notice a slight initial gain. That's great, so don't worry.

You should, however, have an idea of what your starting point is. If you opted for the keto diet solely to lose weight, you'll be able to track your progress. But don't become a slave to the scale. The occasional weigh-in, perhaps once a week, is enough.

What About Your Favorite Meals?

Perhaps the very thought of giving up your favorite foods has prevented you from getting started on the keto way of life. Relax. The truth is, for every dish that you love and can't live without (yes, that includes cheesecake and mashed potatoes!), you can easily find a low-carb substitute that is just as tasty.

First, let's consider items at your market labeled "low carbohydrate." Labels are frustratingly deceiving, and you'd have to be a nutritional expert to understand them. All too frequently, off-the-shelf low carb products have simply substituted sugar for carbs, so don't fall for that bit of deceit. You need to learn to read labels with the diligence that you'd read your wealthy uncle's will, but your best bet is to stay away from these products and simply find healthier substitutes. The same goes for anything labeled "low fat" which inevitably means added sugars.

Craving a taco? Use a lettuce wrap instead of a taco shell. Do you want rice or mashed potatoes? Grate or rice a cauliflower, and you won't be able to tell the difference. Can't give up your favorite pasta dish? Turn a zucchini into "zoodles" by slicing it or using a spiral cutter and enjoy your pasta. You absolutely have to have your favorite dessert? On the keto diet, you can. Just bake with almond flour and use unsweetened applesauce and/or avocado to create some sweet smoothness.

Learn about coconut oil, which can be used as a butter substitute in sautéing, frying, and baking. Coconut oil has incredible health benefits, especially for Type-2 diabetics.

On the keto diet, you'll be able to enjoy all your favorite meals, only better.

Always Stay Hydrated

The keto diet tends to lower your insulin level, so your kidneys may be excreting more liquid than usual. Be sure to drink plenty of water.

Condiments Can Be the Enemy

Don't assume condiments don't count on a diet. On the keto diet, they most certainly do. Ketchup is filled with sugar. Not all salad dressings are equal. Read the label, and never opt for the "fat-free" version. They have merely substituted sugar for fat.

Ordering salads when eating out is one of your best options, but beware of the dressing that the restaurant serves. Either ask about the ingredients, or better, bring your own salad dressing. Don't hesitate to do that, even in a posh eatery where the Maître d' might be horrified at the sight of you pulling salad dressing out of your bag.

4 Minute Keto

Keep Track of Your Ketone Level

It's especially important to remain aware of how your body is responding to the keto diet at the start of the diet. You can do so by doing a simple urine test. You can also purchase a blood ketone meter. It is recommended to perform the test early in the morning.

Friends and Family Can Be Annoying

Those nearest and dearest to you may not always understand what you are doing. When eating as a group, they may put subtle pressure on you to "just try a bite," or "one slice of cake won't kill you." Or worse, "but I cooked it especially for you!"

It will take resolve to stick to your diet. It may help to fill up on keto-friendly snacks before you sit down and eat. Enjoy some nuts, an avocado, or just a leg of chicken *before* you eat, and you will be far less tempted.

Celebrate!

Celebratory occasions, especially if you're the guest of honor, can be a huge hurdle. When the gang at the office or your parents enter a room with a cake yelling "Surprise!" on your birthday, it's hard to refuse. So, try being a bit sneaky, instead.

By all means gush over the offering. You are expected to do that. You can even help cut slices. Then, discover a sudden and irresistible urge for coffee, which you verbalize loudly and clearly. Gently remove yourself from the center of activity to get coffee for yourself and anyone else. By the time anyone notices, hopefully they've missed the fact that you haven't eaten anything.

Traveling

Traveling while on the keto diet can be a challenge, so be prepared. Pack a personal blender with some avocados and bananas for a few quick and healthful smoothies. Pack some anchovies or tuna for protein.

Eating Out

Eating out isn't as difficult as you may think. Even fast-food places have salads these days. In any restaurant, stick to meat and vegetables and forego the potatoes and noodles.

You can even navigate the tricky maze in a Chinese restaurant. While abstaining from rice, you can enjoy the following: clear soups, steamed fish with vegetables, egg foo young, stir-fried dishes, Mu Shu without the wrappers. These are just a few suggestions. Ask your server if your meal can be prepared without cornstarch which is frequently used as a thickener.

Even if you end up in a fast food place that doesn't have salad, simply toss the buns from your burger and just eat the meat. You can do the same at a friend's house or at a BBQ.

Exercise

The keto diet will build muscle mass and give you added energy. Don't forget to incorporate exercise into your daily routine. It can be as simple as walking more, taking the stairs, or joining a gym.

4 Minute Keto

How Long Should You Diet For?"

The amount of time spent on the diet can vary and should be discussed with your doctor. Many people who use the ketogenic diet for weight loss remain on the diet for several weeks, until they have achieved a goal, then they turn to a paleo diet or other maintenance eating. You do not want to lose weight only to return to your old eating habits.

If you are on the ketogenic diet for medical or therapeutic reasons, check with your doctor to ascertain if you should remain on the diet for a longer period of time.

4 Minute Keto

Turn your body into a lean, mean, fat-burning machine

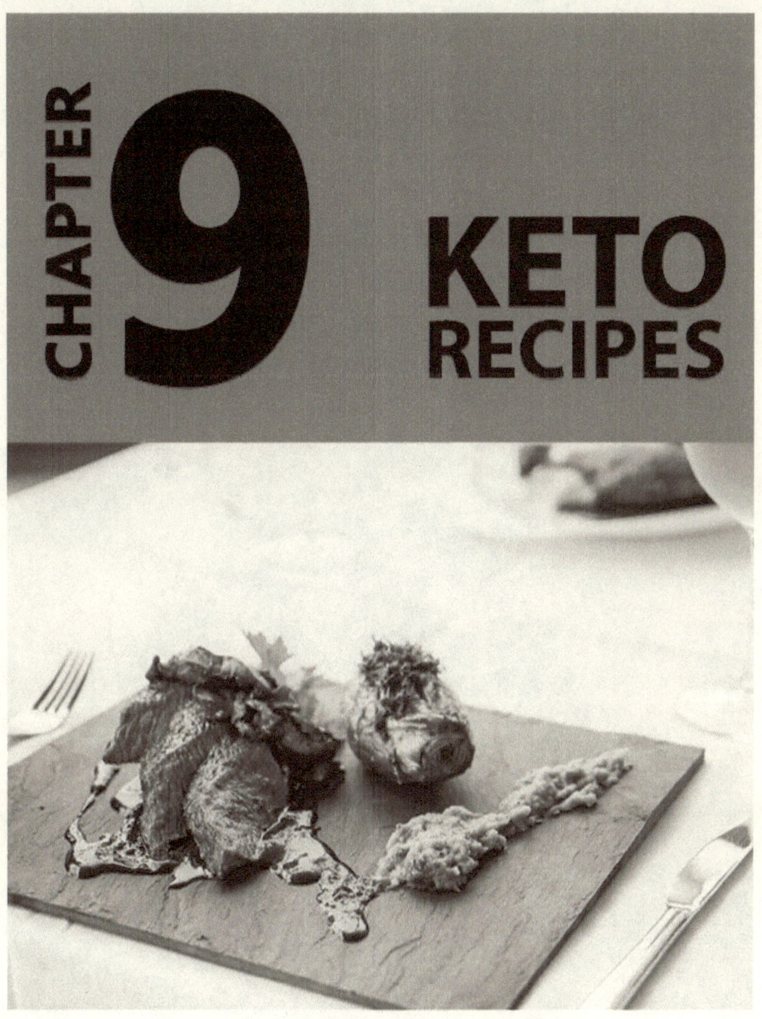

Chapter 9: Keto Recipes

You can take your favorite recipes and turn them "keto." Below are a few recipes to show you how easy it is.

4 Minute Keto

Turn your body into a lean, mean, fat-burning machine

Don't be trapped into believing that a particular recipe has to be for breakfast or lunch or dinner. Eat what you like, when you like. It wouldn't be the first time I've sat down to bacon and eggs for dinner!

My Go-To Breakfast

This is my favorite breakfast. Though of course you can have it for lunch or dinner instead. Around five minutes to prepare, less than $5 total cost, thoroughly keto and totally delicious.

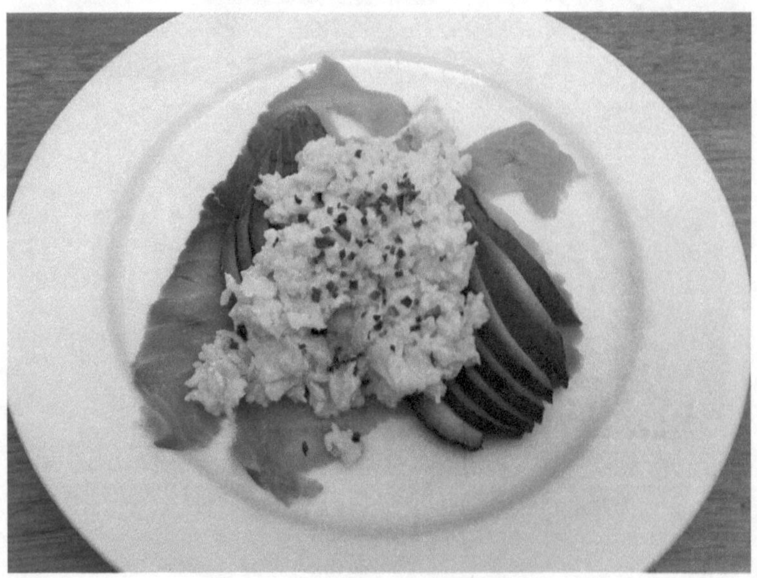

4 Minute Keto

Turn your body into a lean, mean, fat-burning machine

Ingredients

> 3 large, free-range eggs
> 2 slices of smoked salmon
> Knob of butter
> Half an avocado
> Chopped chives (optional)

Directions

Halve and then quarter an avocado and discard the seed. Peel the quarters and fan or slice two of them. Wrap the other two in cling wrap and keep them in the fridge for tomorrow.

Place the two slices of smoked salmon on a plate and the fanned avocado on top.

Heat a decent knob of butter (real butter, not an artificial "spreadable" full of chemicals and other stuff) on a non-stick frypan on high heat.

In the meantime, break two or three eggs into a bowl and whisk briskly with a fork.

Spread the melted butter over the pan, reduce the heat to medium and pour the scrambled egg mix on top.

Using a wooden spoon, continually scrape the egg mix from the outside of the pan towards the center until it's all cooked.

Scrape onto the avocado and sprinkle with chives if desired. (The chives make it look like a "bought one.")

4 Minute Keto

Note that there is no toast. The smoked salmon forms the base.

The Original High Protein Weight Watchers Breakfast

For pretty much the simplest possible, fully keto breakfast, it's hard to go past boiled eggs.

I have two, but you should have however many it takes to get you through to lunch time.

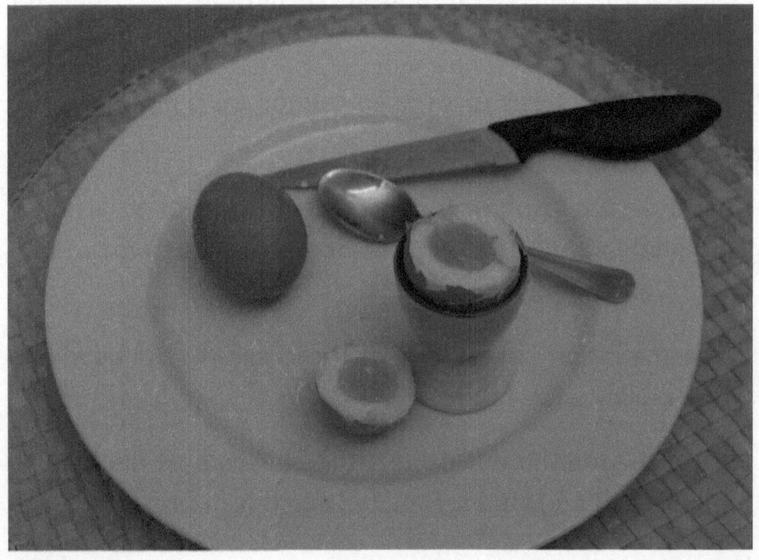

Ingredients

Large, free-range eggs.

Directions

Fill a saucepan with enough water to float the eggs and bring to the boil.

Using a teaspoon, lower the eggs gently into the boiling water.

Remove the eggs after six to seven minutes, depending on their size.

Hint
Run each egg briefly under cold water to make the shells less hot to handle.

If desired, add salt and pepper to taste (I don't).

Remove the tops with a serrated knife and eat with the teaspoon.

Cauliflower Rice and Zoodles

Two of the most important keto recipes are the simple cauliflower rice and "zoodles." They couldn't be easier to prepare. People can get frustrated on the keto diet when they crave pasta and rice. These two recipes definitely satisfy those cravings; they taste just like the real thing. The zoodles can be used for any pasta dish.

4 Minute Keto

Turn your body into a lean, mean, fat-burning machine

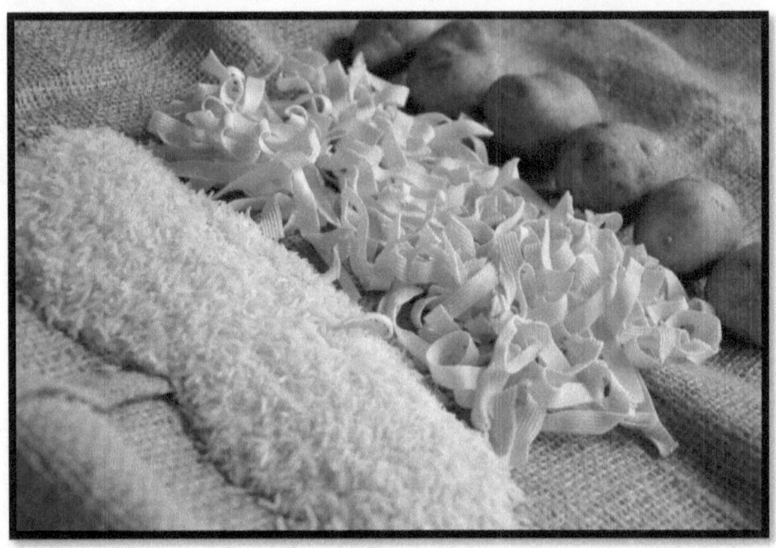

The recipe for Cauliflower Rice can be found on page 86 and the recipe for Zoodles on page 88.

Omelet Muffins

Make plenty of these ahead of time. They'll go fast.

Ingredients

> 1 tbsp. butter
>
> 10 eggs
>
> Salt and pepper to taste
>
> ½ cup diced ham
>
> ¼ cup drained spinach
>
> ¼ cup diced onion
>
> ¼ cup chopped red bell pepper
>
> ¼ cup shredded Pepper Jack cheese

Directions

Preheat the oven to 350 degrees.

4 Minute Keto

Coat a muffin pan with non-stick spray.

Whisk the eggs, then stir in the remaining ingredients.

Fill the muffin pan with the mixture

Bake for 25 minutes.

Nutritional Facts: Calories 155; carb. 2 g; fat 10 g; protein 12.5 g.

Breakfast Casserole

This is a delicious casserole everyone can enjoy. It will leave you satisfied until lunch. Or have it for lunch and be satisfied until dinner!

Ingredients

    10 eggs
    ¼ cup whipping cream
    1 cup ricotta cheese
    1 diced onion
    Salt and pepper to taste
    1 package thawed frozen spinach
    1 cup sliced mushrooms
    1 lb. crumbled sausage meat

Directions

Preheat oven to 350 degrees.

Whisk the eggs, whipping cream, ricotta cheese and onion well

Season with salt and pepper.

Add the spinach, mushrooms, and crumbled sausage.

Bake for 30 minutes.

Home Made Onion and Sage Pork Sausages

You can make these as sausages, form them into patties for keto bunless burgers or create small meatballs for a quick snack. Make as much as you like and freeze what you don't eat.

Ingredients

1 lb (450 gm) of ground pork
2 cloves of garlic, finely chopped
1 medium onion, finely chopped
2 tablespoons of olive oil
2 tablespoons of chopped sage
1 teaspoon of sea salt

Directions

Preheat the oven to 400 F (200 C).

Combine the ground pork with the salt, olive oil, garlic, onion, and sage in a bowl. Divide the mixture into 8 equal amounts and shape each portion to resemble firm sausages, compacting them well to ensure they don't fall apart.

Place each sausage onto a greased baking tray and bake for 15 minutes. Carefully turn and bake for an additional 10-15 minutes until golden.

Home Made Beef Sausages with Caramelized Onion

These beefy sausages have the most delicious sweet, jammy onions running through them and are sure to be a breakfast favorite. The nutritional information is calculated on a serving of two sausages per portion.

Ingredients

- 2 Tablespoons of olive oil (30 ml)
- 1 medium onion (110 g), finely sliced
- 2 Tablespoons of balsamic vinegar (30 ml)
- 1 lb ground beef (450 g)
- 2 Tablespoons of fresh thyme (6 g), picked leaves
- 1 teaspoon salt (5 g)
- Dash of freshly ground black pepper

Directions

Preheat the oven to 400 F (200 C).

Heat the olive oil over low heat and gently fry the onions until softened. The onions will eventually caramelize. Add the balsamic vinegar and cook until all the liquid has evaporated and you are left with jammy, sweet onions. Allow the onions to cool slightly and chop them into small pieces.

Combine the ground beef with the salt, pepper, thyme leaves and the finely chopped onion mixture in a bowl. With clean hands, divide the mixture into 8 equal amounts and shape each portion into firm, round sausage patties, compacting them well to ensure they won't fall apart.

4 Minute Keto

Place each sausage onto a greased baking tray and bake for 15 minutes. Carefully turn them and bake for an additional 10-15 minutes. Alternatively, you could heat a tablespoon of olive oil in a pan and gently fry them over a medium heat on all sides for 10-15 minutes. (If in doubt about doneness, simply break a piece off one end to ensure it is no longer pink.)

Nutrition Facts Per Serve: 377 calories; 2 g sugar; 31 g fat; 3 g carbohydrates; 19 g protein.

Keto Pancakes

Serve these pancakes with butter and sugar-free syrup or with berries.

Ingredients

> 1 ¼ cup almond flour
> 2 tbsp. honey
> Dash of salt
> 1 tsp. baking powder
> 1 tsp. cinnamon
> 6 beaten eggs
> ¼ cup plain Greek yogurt
> 3 tbsp. melted butter
> 1 tsp. lemon extract

Directions

Stir the flour, baking powder, and cinnamon in a bowl.

Combine the eggs, honey, yogurt, lemon extract and butter in another bowl.

Slowly stir the egg mixture into the flour mixture.

4 Minute Keto

Use two tablespoons of batter and drop on a hot griddle.

Cook for 4 minutes, then flip and cook for another 2 minutes.

Continue until all batter has been used.

Nutritional Information: 413 calories; 34 g fat; 18.4 g carbohydrates; 16.3 g protein.

Almond Bread

Freshly baked almond bread is a fabulous Keto substitute for store bought bread. It can be used in many Keto recipes.

It's best toasted in the oven, as it can be a bit too crumbly for the toaster.

Ingredients

2 eggs
1 cup of almond flour
1.5 teaspoons of baking powder
3 tablespoons of olive oil
1 teaspoon of mustard powder
1 teaspoon of sea salt
1 teaspoon of gluten-free instant yeast mixed with 1 tablespoon of tepid water

Directions

Preheat the oven to 350 F (180 C).

Combine the eggs, almond flour, baking powder, mustard powder, salt, olive oil and the yeast mixture.

Mix well to form a sticky dough.

Place the mixture into a small greased baking tin (3.5 in x 8 in / 9 cm x 20 cm) and smooth on top.

Bake for 30 minutes.

Carefully tip out of the baking tin and slice into 4 bread slice-sized squares, essentially making 4 thick slices (something like a focaccia or flat bread).

Use as toast, to make French toast, or as sandwich bread.

Roasted Tomatoes and Mushrooms

Ingredients

     1 tablespoon of olive oil
     1 large flat or portabella mushroom
     2 slices of tomato
     1 clove of garlic, peeled and finely chopped
     1 tablespoon of basil, finely shredded
     salt and pepper to taste
     1 slice of almond bread (see recipe on page 79)

Directions

Heat olive oil in a pan and fry the mushroom until softened and cooked through. Season and set aside.

Fry the tomato slices with the garlic until soft.

Place the cooked mushroom and tomatoes onto the almond bread. Slice and scatter the shredded basil on top.

Season with salt and pepper to taste and serve.

4 Minute Keto

Apple Red Cabbage

Cabbage is a great vegetable to have on keto. This red cabbage side dish is yummy.

Ingredients

8 slices of bacon, cut into pieces

1 large diced onion

1 peeled and sliced apple

2 cup chicken broth

3 tbsp. red cider vinegar

2 tbsp. coconut palm sugar or sugar substitute, such as Splenda

1 tsp. ground cloves

½ tsp. allspice

½ tsp. nutmeg

Salt and pepper to taste

1 shredded red cabbage

Directions

Fry the bacon in a skillet until crispy.

Add the onion and sauté for 5-6 minutes.

Stir in the broth, sugar, vinegar, spices, salt and pepper.

Add the cabbage and cook on low for 45 minutes.

Nutrition Facts: 160 calories; 7.8 g fat; 16 g carbohydrates; 4 g protein.

4 Minute Keto

Tuna and Tomato Bruschetta

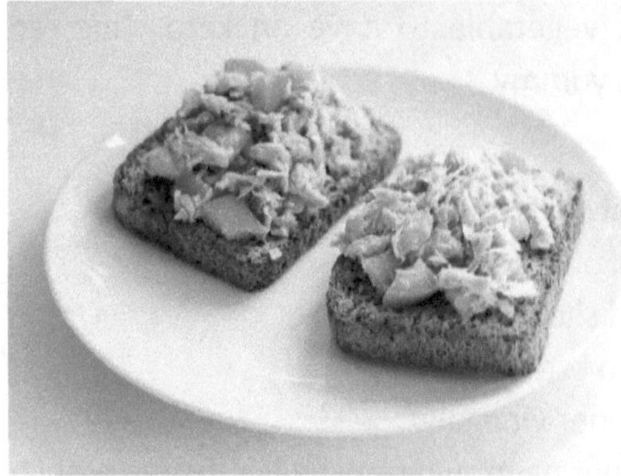

This is a delicious ketogenic twist on the Italian classic.

It's a good lunchtime or appetizer recipe as the bruschetta is so tasty and easy to make. It makes the perfect starter for an Italian-inspired meal, and shows your family and friends that keto doesn't have to be boring! The freshness of the tomato offsets the oiliness of the tuna and you can add some fresh herbs and seasonings to boost the flavor even more.

Ingredients

> 4 slices of keto bread
> 4 tablespoons (60 ml) of extra virgin olive oil
> 1 6 oz (70 gm) can of tuna, drained and flaked
> 1 finely diced tomato
> 1 tablespoon (15 ml) of lemon juice
> 1/4 cup of finely chopped parsley
> Salt and pepper to taste

4 Minute Keto

Turn your body into a lean, mean, fat-burning machine

Directions

Toast the keto bread and spread most of the olive oil over the slices.

Mix the tuna, tomato, lemon juice, and parsley in a bowl and season with salt and pepper.

Serves 4 as a snack or 2 as a lunch.

Nutrition Facts Per Serve: 343 calories; 1 g sugar; 30 g fat; 4 g carbohydrates; 16 g protein.

Variations

Use salmon instead of tuna.
Add chopped, pitted olives to the mix.
Top with grilled bacon!

Cinnamon Granola

Store-bought granola usually has a high sugar content. Try this instead.

Ingredients

1 cup chopped walnuts
½ cup shredded coconuts
¼ cup sliced almonds
2 tbsp. sunflower seeds
½ tsp. cinnamon
1 tbsp. coconut palm sugar
1 tbsp. melted butter

Directions

Preheat the oven to 375 degrees.

4 Minute Keto

Combine the walnuts, shredded coconut, sliced almonds, and sunflower seeds.

Add cinnamon and coconut palm sugar and stir into the nut mixture.

Spread the mixture in a single layer on a baking sheet.

Drizzle with the melted butter.

Bake for 20 minutes.

Nutrition Facts: 180 calories; 19 g fat; 4.1 g carbohydrates; 4 g protein.

Herbed Omelet with Smoked Salmon

You can enjoy this omelet anytime, but a breakfast of protein and fatty acids gets the day started right.

Ingredients

2 tbsp. butter
2 beaten eggs
1 tsp. tarragon
1 tsp. thyme
Salt and pepper to taste
1 tbsp. butter
2 tbsp. chopped onions
4 very thin tomato slices
2 smoked salmon sliced
1 tsp. capers

Directions
Whisk the eggs and add the tarragon, thyme, salt, and pepper.

4 Minute Keto

Melt the butter in a skillet and add the beaten eggs and chopped onions.

Cook for 3-4 minutes, until the eggs begin to set.

Transfer the omelet to a plate and top with the tomato and salmon slices. Sprinkle with capers.

Nutrition Facts: Calories: 239; fat 15 g; carbohydrates 4 g; protein 22 g.

Cheeseburger Salad

This is your favorite cheeseburger without the bun.

Ingredients

>   1 lb. ground beef
>   Salt and pepper to taste
>   3 cups chopped lettuce
>   1 small diced onion
>   1 sliced tomato
>   ¼ cup shredded cheddar cheese
>   4 tbsp. oil and vinegar dressing

Directions

Fry the ground beef in a skillet for 4 minutes.

Add the onion and cook for another 5 minutes.

Place the beef and onions in a bowl and add the remaining ingredients, except the dressing.

Coat with the salad dressing.

Nutrition Facts: Calories 290; Fat 14 g; Carbohydrates 6; Protein 25 g.

4 Minute Keto

Lemon Garlic Baked Shrimp

Who doesn't like fish with lemon? It's a classic! If you prefer, this dish can be cooked in the oven, but the shrimp look amazing threaded onto skewers and grilled. The peppers add loads of color and you can use any type of mushroom you prefer. Impress your guests at your next dinner party or serve this at the next family barbecue for a Keto-friendly dish the whole family will enjoy.

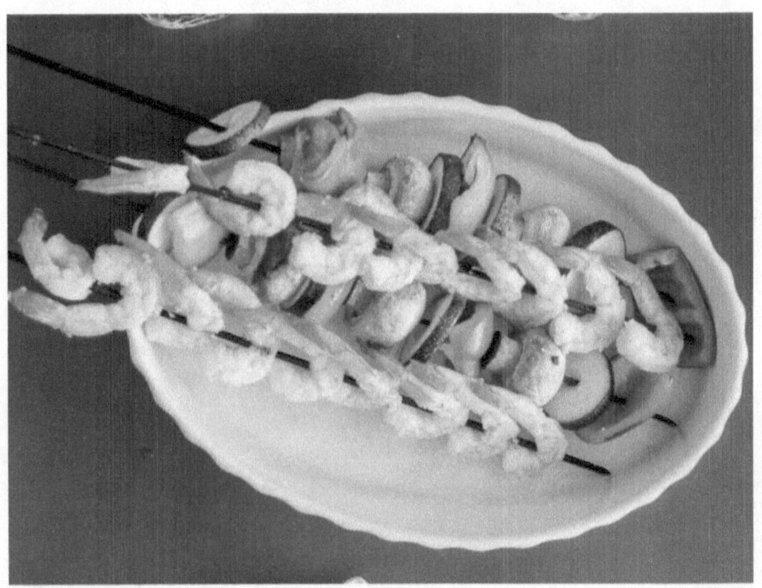

Ingredients

- 1 lb (450 g) shrimp, peeled and deveined
- 8 cloves garlic, minced
- 1/2 Tablespoon lemon juice
- 2 Tablespoons ghee
- 1/2 teaspoon salt
- 1/4 teaspoon black pepper

4 Minute Keto

  2 bell peppers, chopped
  4 mushrooms
  1 zucchini, chopped

Directions

Preheat oven to 400F.

In a bowl, melt the ghee, then add in the minced garlic, salt, and pepper. Divide the mixture in half – save one half of the mixture for serving with.

Dip each shrimp in one half of the mixture and put on skewers.

Place the chopped bell peppers, mushrooms, and zucchini slices on skewers.

Place the skewers on a baking tray and cook the skewers approximately 5 minutes on each side.

Serve with the saved garlic ghee mixture.

Nutrition Facts Per Serve: Calories 400; Sugar 2 g; Fat 17 g; Carbohydrates 9; Protein 43 g.

Cauliflower Rice

This very simple recipe is for basic rice. You can dress it up with vegetables, spices, or stir fry it. Use this anytime you need rice as a side dish or in a recipe.

Ingredients

  1 cauliflower head

Directions

Chop the cauliflower into florets.

4 Minute Keto

Place the florets in a food processor and pulse until you have a rice-like consistency.

Cook the rice in a pan of salted water for 5 minutes.

Nutritional Facts: Calories 21; Carbohydrates 5; Fat 0; Protein 0

Zoodles

These zoodles made from zucchini taste like noodles. A spiralizer is the easiest way to create zoodles, but you can also use a mandolin. Zoodles get soggy very easily, so do not cook for more than 1 minute. Season with butter or shredded cheese.

Ingredients

> 1 zucchini

Directions

Use a spiralizer to create pasta strands.

Bring a pot of salted water to boil and cook the zoodles for 1 minute.

Bacon-Wrapped Chicken

A very decadent and delicious way to enjoy chicken.

Ingredients

> 2 lbs. boneless and skinless chicken breast
> 2 cups chopped spinach
> 1 cup sliced mushrooms
> 1 cup cream cheese
> ½ cup cottage cheese

4 Minute Keto

Turn your body into a lean, mean, fat-burning machine

        Salt and pepper to taste
        12 slices bacon

Directions

Preheat the oven to 375 degrees

Combine the spinach, mushroom, cream cheese and cottage cheese in a bowl.

Season the mixture with salt and pepper.

Use a mallet to flatten the chicken pieces to a 1/2 -inch thickness.

Use a sharp knife to cut pockets in one end.

Spoon the mixture into the pockets.

Wrap two bacon slices around each chicken piece.

Brown the wrapped chicken in a skillet 5 minutes each side.

Place the chicken pieces in a baking dish.

Bake the chicken for 45 minutes. The bacon should be crispy and the chicken done.

Nutrition Facts: Calories 390; Fat 22 g; Carbs 3.9 g; Protein 41 g.

Cobb Salad

This salad is very high in protein. Enjoy.

Ingredients for Dressing

        1 tbsp. olive oil
        1 tbsp. white vinegar

    1 tsp. Dijon mustard
    2 tbsp. diced onion
    Salt and pepper to taste

Ingredients for Cobb Salad

    ¾ cup cubed cooked chicken
    ½ cup diced tomatoes
    ½ cup blue cheese
    2 tablespoons blue cheese
    1 sliced hard-boiled egg
    2 cups chopped greens
    1 sliced avocado
    4 cooked and sliced bacon slices

Directions

Arrange the greens on a plate.

Arrange rows of chicken, diced tomatoes, blue cheese, egg slices, avocado slices and bacon pieces on top of the greens.

Combine all dressing ingredients.

Drizzle the dressing over the salad.

Nutrition facts: Calories 295; Fat 11 g; Carbs 4 g; Protein 22 g.

Slow Cooker Pot Roast

This pot roast is prepared without potatoes or carrots. If you add them, adjust the carbs accordingly.

Ingredients

    2 lb. chuck roast
    Salt and pepper to taste

4 Minute Keto

Turn your body into a lean, mean, fat-burning machine

> 1 tbsp. olive oil
> 2 minced garlic cloves
> 1 chopped onion
> 2 ½ cup beef broth
> ½ cup dry red wine

Directions

Season the roast with salt and pepper.

Salt and pepper the roast.

Heat the olive oil in a skillet and brown the roast on all sides.

Place the roast and remaining ingredients in the slow cooker.

Stir the ingredients to combine.

Cook on low for 6 hours.

Nutrition facts: Calories 242; Fat 12 g; Carbs 9.8 g; Protein 21g.

Spinach and Sausage Soup

This soup is loaded with flavor while remaining very low in carbs.

Ingredients

> 1 lb. spicy crumbled Italian sausage
> 1 tbsp. olive oil
> 1 chopped onion
> 2 sliced carrots
> 1 minced garlic clove
> 2 tbsp. red wine vinegar

4 Minute Keto

½ tsp. oregano
Dash of hot sauce
4 cups chicken broth
½ cup whipping cream
2 cups baby spinach
Salt and pepper to taste

Directions

Heat the olive oil in a skillet and saute the crumbled sausage for 5 minutes, until it is no longer pink.

Transfer the sausage to a plate and drain on a paper towel.

Sauté the onion, garlic, and carrot in the same pan.

Deglaze the pan with the red wine vinegar.

Add the chicken stock, whipping cream, oregano and hot sauce and stir well. Season with salt and pepper.

Simmer the soup for 5 minutes.

Transfer the sausage back into the pan and stir in the spinach.

Cook for 1 minute to allow the spinach to wilt.

Nutrition facts: Calories 137; Fat 7.8 g; Carbs 2 g; Protein 11g.

Tandoori Chicken

Tandoori chicken is all about the spice marinade. Serve it with some cauliflower rice.

4 Minute Keto

Ingredients

2 lbs. chicken thighs

Ingredients for Marinade

1 cup plain yogurt
2 tsp. lemon juice
Salt and pepper to taste
2 tbsp. olive oil
2 minced garlic cloves
1 tsp. chili powder
1 tsp. grated fresh ginger
1 tsp. garam masala
½ tsp. cumin

Directions

With a sharp knife, cut several slits into the chicken thighs.

Season the chicken with salt and pepper and drizzle with the lemon juice.

Combine the remaining ingredients in a large bowl.

Place the chicken in the bowl and coat thoroughly.

Refrigerate up to 24 hours. The longer you marinate, the more flavor is absorbed.

Preheat the oven to 375 degrees.

Line a baking sheet with aluminum foil and layer the chicken on top.

Bake for about 45 – 50 minutes, until the skin is nice and crispy.

4 Minute Keto

Nutrition facts: Calories 145; Fat 5.8 g; Carbs 2.3 g; Protein 17g.

Beef Wellington

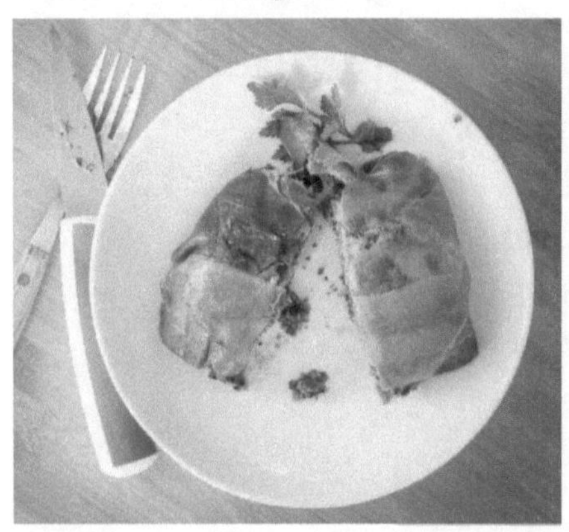

Beef Wellington is a dish that you will sometimes find on the menu at an up-market restaurant. It's also a great dinner to make at home as a romantic dinner for two, a dinner party or a special occasion such as someone's birthday. The problem from a Keto point of view is the pastry, but this clever recipe gives you beef wellington wrapped in prosciutto instead, giving it the same look, but boosting the flavor even more. The mushrooms give the meat a wonderful coating. This dish is best if you use fillet or another high-end cut of beef.

This recipe includes duxelles. Here is Wikipedia's definition:

Duxelles is a finely chopped mixture of mushrooms or mushroom stems, onions or shallots, herbs such as thyme or parsley, and black pepper, sautéed in butter and reduced to a paste. Cream is sometimes used as well, and some recipes add a dash of madeira or sherry. It is a basic preparation used in stuffings and sauces or as a garnish. Duxelles can also be filled into a pocket of raw pastry and baked as a savory tart.

4 Minute Keto

Turn your body into a lean, mean, fat-burning machine

Ingredients for the Duxelles

- 3 large button mushrooms
- 1 Tablespoon (10 g) onions, chopped
- 1 teaspoon (3 g) garlic powder
- 1/2 teaspoon (3 g) salt
- 2 Tablespoons (30 ml) olive oil

Other Ingredients

- 1 9-ounce (252 g) filet mignon
- 8 thin slices of prosciutto (or 4 ham slices)
- 1 Tablespoon (14 g) yellow mustard
- 1/2 Tablespoon (7 g) salt
- 2 Tablespoons (30 ml) olive oil to cook in

Directions

Preheat oven to 400 F (200 C).

Make the duxelles by blending the mushrooms, onions, garlic, salt, and olive oil together until pureed.

Then heat the mixture in a pan for 10 minutes on medium heat.

Place a large piece of cling wrap onto the counter and place the slices of prosciutto side-by-side (overlapping slightly) to form a rectangular layer.

Spread the duxelles over the prosciutto layer.

Sprinkle the 1/2 Tablespoon of salt over the filet mignon.

Pan-sear the filet mignon in 2 Tablespoons of olive oil.

4 Minute Keto

Spread the 1 Tablespoon of mustard on the seared filet mignon and place in the middle of the prosciutto and duxelles layer.

Use the cling wrap to wrap the prosciutto around the filet mignon. Then wrap the cling wrap around the package to secure it. Use a second piece of cling wrap to pull the prosciutto-wrapped package tighter together. Place in fridge for 15 minutes.

Remove the cling wrap from the refrigerated prosciutto-wrapped beef and place on a greased baking tray.

Bake for 20-25 minutes (it should be pink when you cut into it).

To serve, carefully cut the Beef Wellington in half.

Nutrition facts: Calories 580; Fat 50 g; Carbs 2 g; Protein 30 g.

Curried Lamb

Filled with exotic spices, this curry dish is perfect with keto rice.

Ingredients

- 2 lbs. lamb meat
- 1 tbsp. olive oil
- 1 diced onion
- 3 minced garlic cloves
- ½ tsp. grated ginger
- ½ to. turmeric
- ½ tsp. curry powder

4 Minute Keto

Turn your body into a lean, mean, fat-burning machine

    ½ tsp. garam masala

    2 cups beef stock

    1 cup plain Greek yogurt

    1 tsp. lemon juice

Directions

Cut the lamb meat into small pieces

Sauté the onion in the olive oil for 5 minutes, then add the garlic, ginger, turmeric, curry powder and garam masala. Stir for another 5 minutes.

Add the meat and brown it for 10 minutes.

Pour in the beef stock and simmer for 40 minutes.

Remove from heat and stir in the yogurt and lemon juice.

Nutrition Facts: Calories 329; Fat 17 g; Carbs 9.1 g; Protein 36 g.

Cheddar Biscuits

These tasty biscuits are great anytime. They freeze well, so keep them handy.

Ingredients

    2 cups almond flour

    1 cup shredded cheddar cheese

    1 cup coconut oil

    1 cup cream cheese

    3 eggs

    2 tsp. baking powder

    1 tsp. baking soda

    Dash of salt

4 Minute Keto

Directions

Preheat oven to 325 degrees.

Cover a baking sheet with aluminum foil.

Place the flour and the cheese in a food processor and pulse to a grainy consistency.

Add the baking powder and baking soda.

Heat the cream cheese and coconut oil in a small pan and warm until they melt. Stir to a creamy smoothness.

Whisk the eggs and add the salt.

Stir the flour mixture into the egg mixture and stir until a dough forms.

Use a tablespoon to drop the dough onto the baking sheet.

Bake for 25 minutes.

Allow the biscuits to cool for slicing.

Nutrition Facts: Calories 106; Fat 11.1 g; Carbs 2 g; Protein 3.9 g.

Really Simple Keto Dinner

Sometimes, I just can't be bothered cooking anything that requires the complexity of a recipe.

Here's a formula that requires no preparation and minimal cooking time, but is satisfying, delicious and totally keto.

4 Minute Keto

The "formula" is one piece of protein and two or three vegetables, cooked simply and selected from the following table:

Protein	Green Veg	Yellow Veg	Other
Grass-fed beef steak (rump, sirloin, rib-eye etc.)	Broccoli	Carrot	Mushroom
Salmon fillet	Beans	Pumpkin	
Lamb chops	Peas	Squash	
White fish	Spinach		
Pork (fillet, chop, loin etc.)	Zucchini		
Chicken breast	Brussel sprouts		
Butterflied chicken quarter	Silverbeet		
English pork sausage			

Clearly, there are many combinations that you can use here to create variety.

I've included the butterflied chicken quarter because a lot of butchers sell butterflied chicken (I even know of one that labels it "run-over rooster") often with an added spice such as lemongrass. It's easily divided into four – two each of breast + wing and thigh + drumstick. Absolutely delicious!

4 Minute Keto

Turn your body into a lean, mean, fat-burning machine

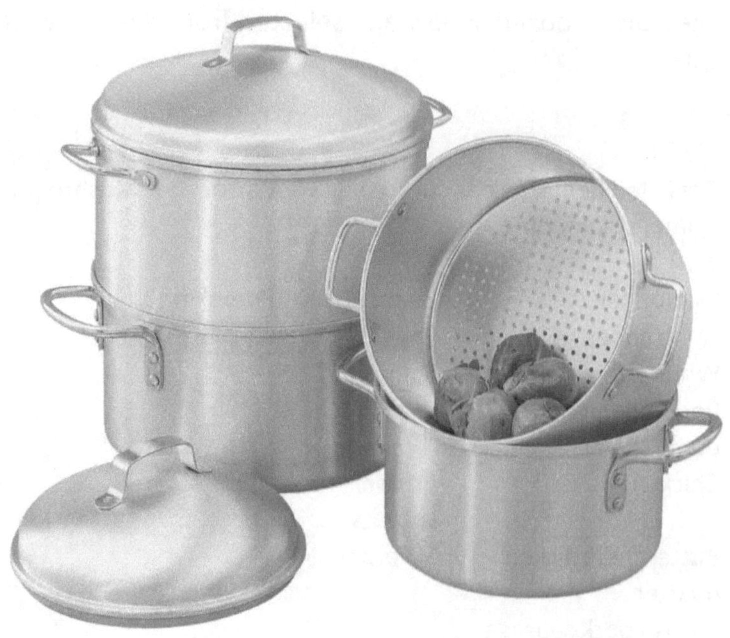

Keep the cooking totally basic. Broil or grill the protein or cook it in a non-stick frypan with a little extra virgin olive oil or coconut oil. Other than mushrooms, zucchini, spinach and silver-beet, simply steam the vegetables.

Mushrooms and zucchini can be sliced and done in the frypan.

Spinach and silver-beet can be wilted in the frypan. Just add to hot oil and turn over several times with tongs. It will reduce to about one-fifth of its original volume.

Here's how the timing works for me.

4 Minute Keto

Let's say I decide to cook sirloin steak, broccoli, pumpkin and mushroom for dinner.

I put water in the steamer's saucepan and set it on the stove to boil.

I cut florets off the broccoli, cut a slice of pumpkin and remove the skin and seeds. If it's a big enough slice, cut it in half.

I cut a decent sized field mushroom into slices or wedges.

Put a non-stick frypan onto the stove top at medium heat, add a couple of slurps of extra virgin olive oil, add the sirloin steak and rub both sides in the oil.

When the water boils, add the broccoli and pumpkin to the steamer.

When the steak is done to your liking on one side, turn it over and add the mushroom slices or wedges to the frypan. Turn them after a few minutes so they are nicely cooked on each side.

When the steak is done, everything else will be too.

Serve the steak on a plate with the mushrooms on top and the two vegetables next to it.

Don't add mustard or any kind of sauce. It just detracts from the flavor of the steak. Under no circumstances add a sprig of parsley!

Enjoy this plain, simple ketogenic meal with a minimum of fuss.

4 Minute Keto

Don't be overly concerned about portion sizes. The idea is to consume a meal that doesn't leave you either hungry or over full.

Experiment until you get that right, whether it takes two steaks or half of one. And then add the right amount of vegetable to see you through to bed time.

4 Minute Keto

Chapter 10: Keto Diet Conclusion

Congratulations. You've mastered the ketogenic diet. You've lost weight, feel better, look fabulous, and are enjoying an abundance of energy. You've put a lot of effort into improving your health, so what happens when you've reached your goal? Should you abandon the keto diet now?

It's a hard fact that maintaining your weight loss can actually be more difficult than losing that weight in the first place. Returning to your old, bad eating habits may be all too tempting. In addition, when you discontinue the keto diet, your metabolism is likely to slow down, making weight maintenance more difficult.

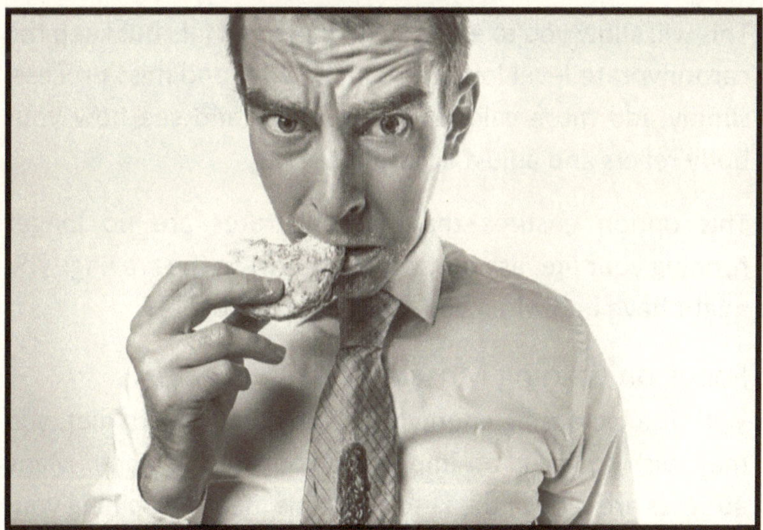

You certainly don't want to lose momentum and return to the unhealthy, Western sugar and carbohydrate swamp,

4 Minute Keto

with your lost weight returning. The options below are undoubtedly best at maintaining your current state of health.

Your Options

Consider your options *before* you stop the keto diet. Have a plan in place and execute it. Since the keto diet provides you with many options, it will be easier to adjust to a maintenance style.

Continue Keto

Continue on the keto diet that has been successful for you but consume more food. Not different, high-carb foods, but the same foods you ate on the diet, in somewhat larger quantities. You'll be eating more calories.

This will allow you to eat more protein and fats but keep the carbohydrate level low. This can be a hit and miss process; simply add more calories to your diet and see how your body reacts and adjust accordingly.

This option ensures that carbohydrates are no longer running your life, as you won't suffer from the cravings you might have had when you started the keto diet.

Focus on Gaining Muscle

With the increasing energy you enjoy on the keto diet, you may wish to focus on improving your muscle tone. Many athletes are fans of the keto diet. This means retaining your low body fat but adding muscle and definition. Strong muscles help strengthen bone density and keep you strong as you age.

4 Minute Keto

The best way to gain strong muscles is to consume more calories in the form of lean proteins. This option is difficult to maintain unless you also include a resistance training exercise program.

Remain on Low Carb but not on Keto

When you use the keto diet to lose weight, your carbohydrate restrictions are fairly strict. You can still maintain your weight with a low carb diet, but not as rigid as keto. There are many healthy beans and legumes you can enjoy by adding a few more carbs to your diet.

How much more carbs is very individual, because every body is different. Add a few cups of beans, lentils, or another serving of carrots to your diet each week and see how your body reacts. If you continue to maintain your goal weight, you're on the right track. Add 10 grams of carbohydrates a week until you are satisfied with the results.

The advantage of this option is that it allows you to eat good, healthy foods that were off limits on the keto diet. Having a greater variety of foods from which to choose will make it easier to maintain your weight.

If you find yourself gaining weight, simply cut down on the added carbs just a bit.

Use Intermittent Fasting

Intermittent fasting gives you additional options. Remember that fasting forces your body to burn fat.

Here are some ways you can fast intermittently:

4 Minute Keto

1. Eat what you want for 5 days, then fast for 2 days.

2. Eat two meals a day instead of three or four, providing for a longer period where you are not consuming food.

When you begin to embrace keto, you will be enjoying all the benefits of healthy eating. By continuing to consume fewer carbohydrates as a lifestyle, your body will remain sleek and strong. You will also be providing it with ammunition to ward off many chronic diseases.

4 Minute Keto

Chapter 11: Start Exercising

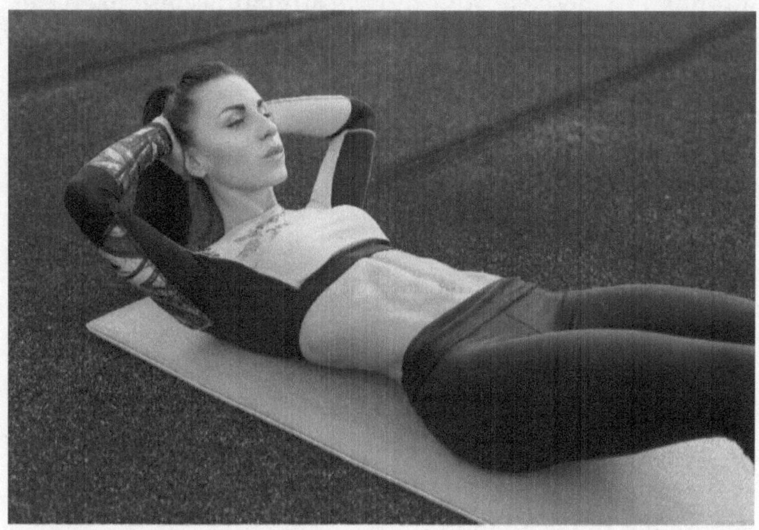

Types of Exercise

While the Keto diet will help you to burn fat and lose weight, exercise will both speed up the process and firm and tone your musculature.

There are three types of exercise that you need to undertake.

HIIT

HIIT stands for High Intensity Interval Training. Basically, it means short bursts of intense exercise, intended to raise your heart and lung rates.

4 Minute Keto

Turn your body into a lean, mean, fat-burning machine

Strength

Intended to increase your muscle strength, these exercises work by creating micro tears in the muscle tissue, which then repairs itself stronger than before.

Abs

Notoriously the hardest muscle group to develop, strong abdominals help you sit and stand tall, and minimize the risk of back pain and injury. These exercises will develop the abs while your keto diet strips away tummy flab to expose them.

The 4 Minute Principle

The good news is that you don't need to spend hours at the gym to get these benefits.

Four minutes a day is all it takes.

There are three different sets of the 4-minute exercises. You do the first set on Monday, the second set on Tuesday and the third on Wednesday.

Repeat for Thursday, Friday and Saturday.

Rest and recover on Sunday.

How easy is that?

4 Minute HIIT

Each four-minute HIIT set consists of two exercises.

You do the first exercise for 20 seconds, rest for 10 seconds and repeat. That's one minute.

4 Minute Keto

Turn your body into a lean, mean, fat-burning machine

You do the second exercise for 20 seconds, rest for 10 seconds and repeat. That's two minutes.

Then repeat steps one and two, for a total of four minutes.

If you need to stop before the 20 seconds are up, that's fine. Just wait out the remainder of the 20 seconds plus the 10 seconds rest and then start the next exercise. The idea is to do what you can and gradually get better and better.

Burpees and Butt Kicks

Burpees for 20 seconds
Rest for 10 seconds
Burpees for 20 seconds
Rest for 10 seconds
Butt Kicks for 20 seconds
Rest for 10 seconds
Butt Kicks for 20 seconds
Rest for 10 seconds
Repeat for a total of 4 minutes

Jump Squats and Plank Jacks

Jump Squats for 20 seconds
Rest for 10 seconds
Jump Squats for 20 seconds
Rest for 10 seconds
Plank Jacks for 20 seconds
Rest for 10 seconds
Plank Jacks for 20 seconds
Rest for 10 seconds
Repeat for a total of 4 minutes

4 Minute Keto

Step Ups and Jumping Jacks
Step Ups for 20 seconds
Rest for 10 seconds
Step Ups for 20 seconds
Rest for 10 seconds
Jumping Jacks for 20 seconds
Rest for 10 seconds
Jumping Jacks for 20 seconds
Rest for 10 seconds
Repeat for a total of 4 minutes

Squat Jacks and Mountain Climbers
Squat Jacks for 20 seconds
Rest for 10 seconds
Squat Jacks for 20 seconds
Rest for 10 seconds
Mountain Climbers for 20 seconds
Rest for 10 seconds
Mountain Climbers for 20 seconds
Rest for 10 seconds
Repeat for a total of 4 minutes

4 Minute Strength

The best exercise you can do for upper body strength without equipment is the ever-reliable pushup.

Similarly, you will use squats for developing lower body strength.

4 Minute Keto

Turn your body into a lean, mean, fat-burning machine

Pushups and Squats

Use the same 20 seconds exercise followed by 10 seconds rest protocol as for the 4-minute HIIT session.

> Pushups for 20 seconds
> Rest for 10 seconds
> Pushups for 20 seconds
> Rest for 10 seconds
> Squats for 20 seconds
> Rest for 10 seconds
> Squats for 20 seconds
> Rest for 10 seconds
> Repeat for a total of 4 minutes

Make sure you do good form pushups and squats. Stop if you need to before the 20 seconds are up but aim to complete the full 20 seconds when you can and then work on increasing the number of reps.

When you're ready to ramp your pushup ambition to the next level, be sure to check out:

4 Minute Keto

Turn your body into a lean, mean, fat-burning machine

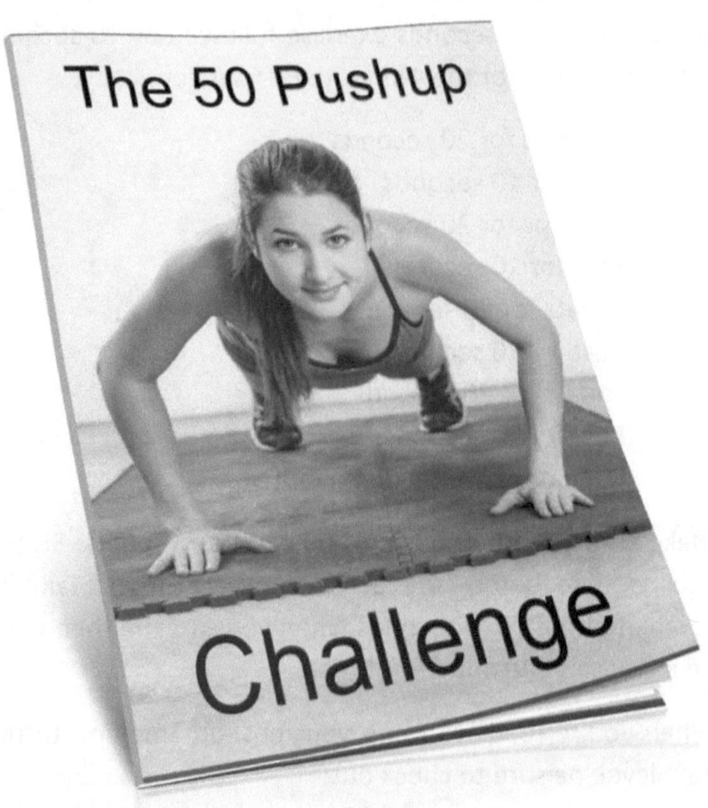

and

4 Minute Keto

Turn your body into a lean, mean, fat-burning machine

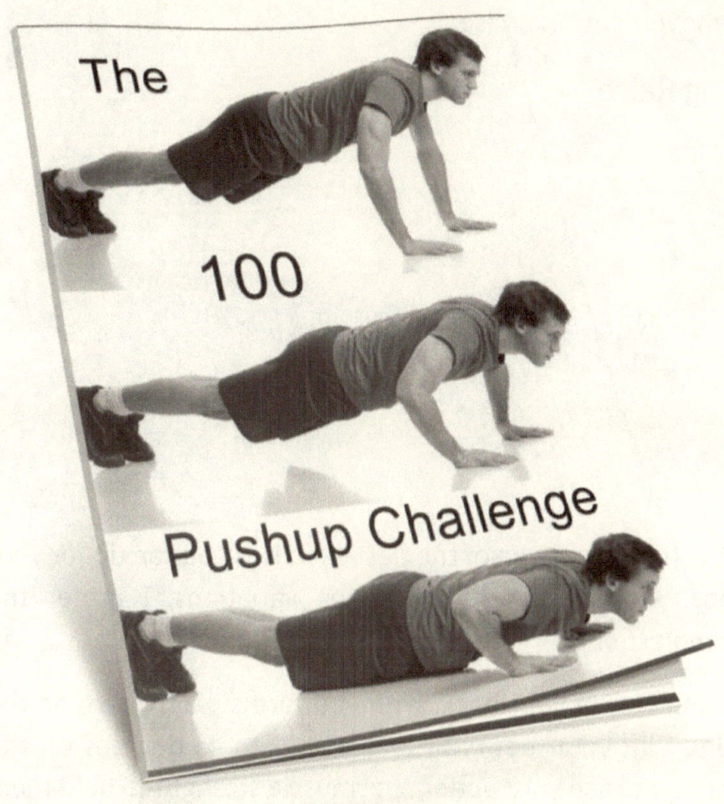

You can get these for free at:

https://agingslowdown.com/pushup-challenge-how-many-can-you-do/

4 Minute Abs

You will do each of these ab exercises for one minute.

4 Minute Keto

Three of them are "hold" exercises and one is a "movement" exercise.

Leg Raise

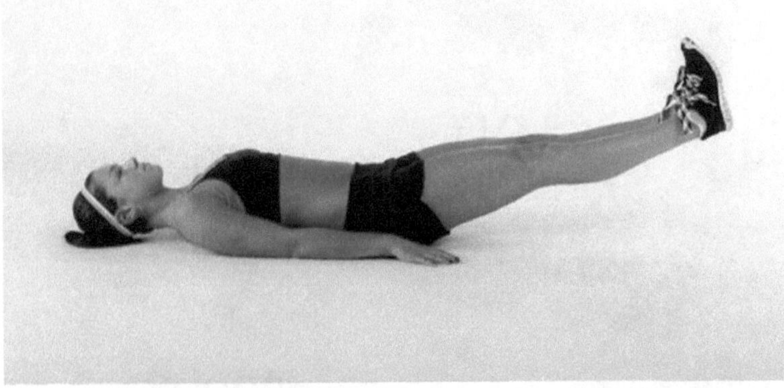

The leg raise is one of the best exercises you can do for your abs. Although there are many variations, I prefer the simplest one.

Lying flat on your back, with your arms palm down on the floor, lift your legs until they are 30 to 45 degrees off the floor and use your abdominal muscle strength to hold them there.

Hold for one minute.

If you can't do that, hold for as long as you can and then lower your legs and rest for the remainder of the minute.

Now you have a goal. Do a bit more each time until you can manage the full minute.

4 Minute Keto

Turn your body into a lean, mean, fat-burning machine

Ramp It Up:

Start off barefoot until you can do the minute easily. Then add heavier and heavier shoes.

Then extend beyond one minute.

Move on to the next exercise immediately.

Sit-up

To do a proper sit-up, you need your ankles immobilized.

Either get a partner to hold them in place or hook them under something heavy like a bed base.

Either cross your arms over your chest or put your hands behind your head.

Sit up until your upper body touches your knees.

Do as many sit-ups as you can in one minute.

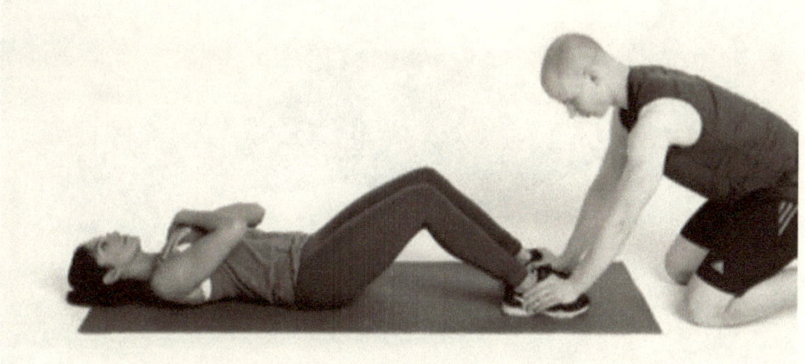

Ramp It Up

Hold a weight against your chest to make your abs work harder.

4 Minute Keto

Plank

The primary muscles the plank works are the erector spinae, the rectus abdominus and the transverse abdominus. The erector spinae is a large muscle that runs up the length of the back. It surrounds your spine and allows you to straighten your back and rotate side to side.

To do a plank, lie on the floor with your body straight and supported on your elbows and toes as shown. Your elbows should be directly under your shoulders.

Keep your body straight. Don't let it sag downwards or bow upwards.

Hold for one minute or as long as you can.

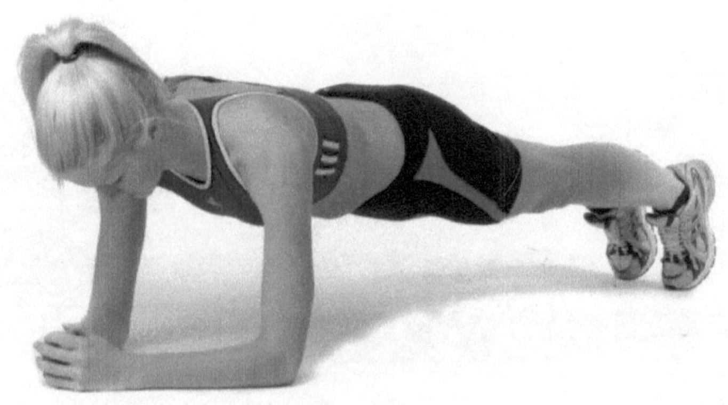

Ramp It Up:
Do an extended plank instead.

4 Minute Keto

Move your elbows forward until they are directly under your ears instead of your shoulders.

This increases the work your abs need to do to hold your body in place.

Or do a regular plank for one minute and then an extended plank for another minute.

Incidentally, I can hold a plank for 5 minutes, but the world record is 8 hours and 1 minute. It was set by Mao Weidong, a Chinese policeman, in 2016.

Oblique Plank

The oblique or side plank targets the often weak muscle called the quadratus lumborum, part of the posterior abdominal wall that plays a prominent role in averting back pain.

Lie on one side of your body and then support yourself on your lower elbow as shown.

Your other arm can be alongside your body or straight up in the air or on your hip. Go with whatever feels comfortable.

4 Minute Keto

Turn your body into a lean, mean, fat-burning machine

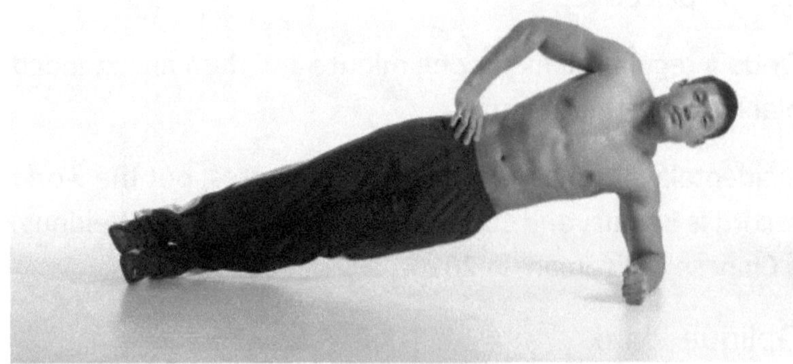

Hold for one minute or as long as you can.

Ramp It Up:

There are several other ways in which you can ramp up your abs exercises and develop a core of steel. To get them for free, sign up at:

https://agingslowdown.com/stay-informed-with-aging-slowdown-offers/

You'll learn variations such as the *Reverse Plank* and the *Superman Plank*.

Stretches

Record Your Progress!

If you don't record your exercise progress (or even lack of it) you are setting yourself up for failure.

I can't over-emphasize how important this is.

4 Minute Keto

Turn your body into a lean, mean, fat-burning machine

Please go to:

https://agingslowdown.com/stay-informed-with-aging-slowdown-offers/

where you can sign up and get the *My Exercise Week* PDF. It's a good idea to <u>print it out</u>.

Fill in your weight, BMI and, if available, your body fat percentage at the start of each week. Then complete your exercise progress every day. Use a pen and complete by hand. It will do wonders for your motivation.

4 Minute Keto

Chapter 12: The Maintenance Phase

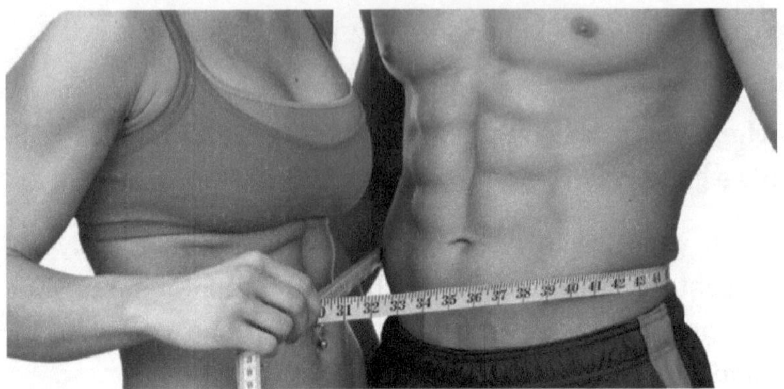

This is what you should do once you've achieved your desired goals.

These could include a specific body weight, BMI or body fat percentage, as well as fitness and wellness levels.

The last thing you want is to fall back into old habits, stack the weight back on and lose the fitness you've achieved.

The simplest maintenance plan is to continue to eat your own home-cooked keto meals for three or four days of the week. For the other three or four days, continue to eat clean, but add some more carbs, such as potato and sweet potato. Include legumes such as beans and peas, but continue to avoid processed food and sugar.

Continue to exercise three days a week and continue to record it, even if you are no longer progressing.

4 Minute Keto

More Health and Fitness Tips

Has eating the Keto way now become a habit and are you looking for different or more intense workouts? Check out my website and download more health and fitness tips at:

https://agingslowdown.com/stay-informed-with-aging-slowdown-offers/

Ramp It Up

How would you like to be one of the few people who can do 100 push-ups without stopping? Or even 50? Go to https://agingslowdown.com/pushup-challenge-how-many-can-you-do/ and download *The 50 Pushup Challenge* and *The 100 Pushup Challenge*.

My Personal Maintenance Plan

I hesitated about including this in this book, because I don't think I'm typical. On the other hand, it really works for me, so perhaps you might get something out of it.

Sunday

Let's start with Sunday.

I regard Sunday as my "day off".

There's a café just around the corner from where I live. They make great coffee, they have an excellent breakfast menu and an ample supply of Sunday newspapers.

I go around there around 10:00am, grab a newspaper and find a nice seat. I don't need to order.

4 Minute Keto

After a couple of minutes, they bring me a mug of extra hot cappuccino and, about five minutes after I've finished it, they deliver their classic breakfast to me, comprising:

> A generous serving of smoky bacon
> Two beautifully poached free-range eggs
> One hash brown
> A bowl of Roma tomatoes in a garlic sauce
> A pile of wilted spinach

(Interestingly, aside from the hash brown, that's essentially keto)

But anyway, I read half the paper while I eat breakfast.

And then about 10 minutes later, they ask if I'd like another coffee.

So another mug of extra hot cappuccino while I finish the paper.

It's an hour to an hour and a half of pure enjoyment.

But here's the thing.

I'm so full from that breakfast that I'm not hungry again until dinner.

I skip lunch entirely.

That's why I said I may not be typical.

But if it works for you, give it a go.

4 Minute Keto

Turn your body into a lean, mean, fat-burning machine

Monday to Saturday

First of all, I walk. Every day. I believe that it's absolutely the best thing you can do.

I'm fortunate to live near a beautiful river. I walk every morning alongside the river to the marina and then back home again. It takes an hour and twenty minutes.

It sets me up for the day, both physically and mentally. By the time I get back home, I have my day planned out.

Diet

I always have a keto breakfast. I just think it's the best start to the day. Frequently, it's my go-to breakfast detailed on page 70 or the traditional bacon (or pork sausages) and eggs.

Sometimes, the simplest possible. Just two soft boiled free-range eggs.

But there are many other options detailed earlier in this book.

Lunch varies.

Sometimes I skip lunch entirely.

Does that make me hungry?

Yes, but I accept the hunger.

Some dieticians give it a label. It's called *Intermittent Fasting*. It's a great way to get into the state of ketosis quickly and also to discipline your body. Get away from the idea that as soon as you feel hungry, you must eat.

4 Minute Keto

Sometimes I have a fruit smoothie. Non-keto, but very satisfying and chock full of vitamins.

I keep plastic containers of sliced fruit in the freezer. Bananas, strawberries, blueberries and mangoes.

4 Minute Keto

The Big Secret

I said this at the start of this book, but it's worth repeating.

It's no secret that the "secret" to losing weight, getting fit, resisting illness and living a long and healthy life is diet and exercise. Yet only a small proportion of the population actually put those two things into practice. As a result, we have overwhelming rates of obesity and a generation of children who, for the first time in history have a lower life expectancy than their parents. How bad is that? I want you to be the exception.

All your meals will be delicious high protein, high fat, low carb. They'll keep your body in a state of ketosis, where instead of metabolising (burning) the glucose in your bloodstream for fuel, it will instead access your stored fat. Your body will become a fat-burning machine. While the Keto diet will help you lose weight by using your body's stored fat as fuel, you'll accelerate this process significantly by exercise. And, of course, exercise will also make you look fitter and leaner, as well as feel (and be) stronger.

But most exercise programs are difficult to maintain. You get started but stop again before it's had a chance to become a habit. Or you just can't find the time to fit your exercise program into your daily routine. That's why I developed the 4 Minute Exercise Program. It consists of a series of exercises, targeting both strength and aerobics, that take just 4 minutes to complete and require no special equipment. The time commitment is low, but the payoff is huge. Easy, right? But the difference between doing something and doing nothing is the biggest difference of all. Reread this book, implement the program and change your life!

4 Minute Keto

Turn your body into a lean, mean, fat-burning machine

The Rest of the Books

The Series

4 Minute Keto is Book 4 in the Fitness Blueprint series:

1. New Year Detox
2. Clean Eating for Weight Loss
3. Beginner's Keto
4. 4 Minute Keto
5. Keto Diet + Intermittent Fasting
6. The Home Workout Bible

Each book can be read stand-alone, but as a series they lead you through a journey, starting with a detox, then learning clean eating and proceeding to the keto diet and exercise to burn fat and become the best you can be.

See the full series at Fitness Blueprint on Amazon.

Other Books

To see all of this author's books, both published and forthcoming titles and to get some free gifts, please sign up at:

https://agingslowdown.com/stay-informed-with-aging-slowdown-offers/

4 Minute Keto

About the Author

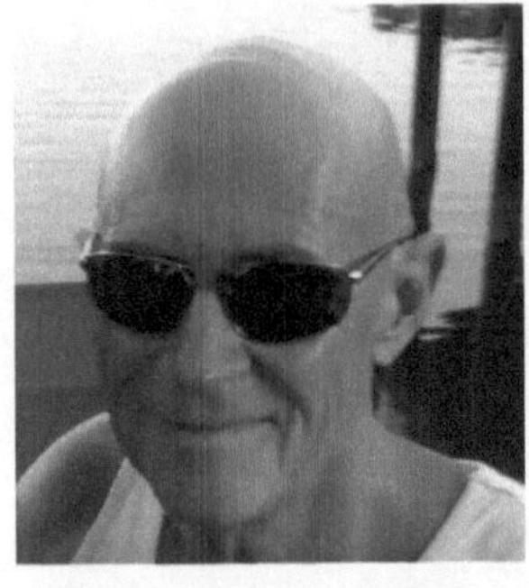 Phil Lancaster is an 80 year old (in 2024) Australian who embraces the Clean Eating and Fitness lifestyle.

He can do 110 pushups without stopping, hold a 5 minute plank, bench press more than his own bodyweight and does 100 km (about 65 miles) bike rides for fun. He weighs the same as he did when he was 18.

He literally never gets a cold or the flu. Not ever. Or hay fever, sniffles, coughing fits or asthma. Or back pain.

And he is a zero contributor to Big Pharma's bottom line.

That's right. He spends nothing on drugs.

No prescribed drugs and no over the counter drugs. He believes that all drugs have undesirable side effects and that most of your medicinal needs can be satisfied by eating the right food and priming your body's natural ability to fight disease and keep you healthy.

He believes that anyone can do the same. You just need to follow the blueprint.

He has 4 children and 5 grandchildren (aged from 15 to 25 years old) and intends to watch them all grow up.